EYE GAZE–BASED OPTIC DISC

by

NILIMA KULKARNI

CONTENTS

ACKNOWLEDGEMENTS

This thesis is result of an exciting and challenging journey of the research. At the end of this journey, I would like to express my gratitude to all the people who contributed and supported for the research. First, I would like to offer my *pranams* to almighty for giving me the opportunity of this research as well as greater inner strength to complete my research work.

My humble pranams to our Chancellor **Sri Mata Amritanandamayi Devi (AMMA)**, who has been a constant source of inspiration. I take this opportunity to sincerely acknowledge the Amrita Vishwa Vidyapeetham for providing necessary infrastructure and resources to carry out the research. I convey my sincere thanks to **Br. Dhanraj** (Director) and **Dr. Rakesh S. G.** (Associate Dean, Amrita School of Engineering, Bengaluru) for their encouragement and support for research work.

I would like to express my deep sense of gratitude to my thesis advisor **Dr. Amudha J.** (Associate Professor and Chairperson, Department of Computer Science and Engineering, Amrita School of Engineering, Bengaluru) for her guidance, endless patience, and continuous encouragement throughout this work. Her unlimited thinking capabilities, flame of curiosity over a problem, and dedication to research have enabled me to gain an insight into the research work. The contents of this thesis are the outcome of prolonged and inspiring discussions that I had with her. Her confidence in me and her inspiring words in times of need have always been great motivating factors for me. I am extremely grateful to her for her excellent guidance and whole-hearted involvement in the research work.

I am grateful to my Doctoral Committee Members **Dr. K.V. Nagaraja** (Convener), **Dr. S. Nandagopalan** (Member External), and **Dr. Sarada Jayan** (Faculty from Minor Area) for offering me suggestions to improve my work and constructive discussions during every review presentation. I would also like to thank **Dr. T.S.B. Sudarshan** (Former Convener) for his suggestions and support for research.

I convey my special thanks to **Salma Jetha** (Patent Coordinator, Amrita Vishwa Vidyapeetham); because of her support only the patent for this research work could be submitted.

I sincerely thank **Dr. Kumar Rajamani** (Manager (Technical)), Robert Bosch Engineering and Business Solutions Ltd, Bengaluru), **Dr. Arcot Sowmya** (Professor, School of Computer Science and Engineering, University of New South Wales, Sydney, Australia), and **Dr. Karthikeyan Vaiapury** (Scientist R&D, TCS Innovation Labs, Chennai) for constructive suggestions and extensive discussions during my Comprehensive Viva-Voce and Open Seminar examinations.

I also thank the staff of SensoMotoric Instruments for providing an SMI eye tracker and support. I sincerely thank to all optometrists and other participants for their enthusiastic participation and support for the research work.

I would like to mention a special thank you to all my Ph.D. course mentors, **Dr. Amudha J., Dr. Deepa Gupta, Dr. Nitu Shrivastva, and Dr. Shrinivas Rao** (ASE Bangalore).

I would like to thank Ms. Chandrika and Ms. Radha D. for their suggestions; my special thanks go to **Ms. Divya K.** for her help and support for the research work. I also thank all the faculty members, non-faculty members, and my fellow research scholar friends of the college for their support during the research work. I also thank to **Mr. Shiv Kumar** for help he provided in editing and proofreading the thesis.

I would like to pay high regards to my husband **Mr. Narendra Rajurkar** for his unlimited support during this research work. He understood my tensions, worries, and always stood beside me in all phases of life. I am able to reach at the end of this research because of his unconditional love and his confidence in me. I specially thank my beloved son, **Master Chinmay Rajurkar**, for his cooperation and patience throughout the period of my study.

Parents' blessings and sibling's wishes always work as good fortune for me. I thank my mother **Mrs. Anuradha Kulkarni** and brother **Mr. Rajendra Kulkarni** for their support, care, love, motivation, understanding, and prayers. I thank my father **Late Mr. Vijay Kulkarni**, whose blessings from above has made me to complete this work successfully.

I also thank my in-laws, especially mother-in-law **Mrs. Indira Rajurkar**, for the help she provided during course work.

Finally, I express my gratitude to one and all who have knowingly or unknowingly, directly or indirectly helped me in the successful completion of this work.

Nilima Kulkarni

LIST OF FIGURES

LIST OF TABLES

LIST OF ABBREVIATIONS AND SYMBOLS

2D	Two-dimensional
3CCD	Three charge-coupled devices
ADHD	Attention-deficit/hyperactivity disorder
AIDS	Acquired immunodeficiency syndrome
ALRIEGA	Automatic labeling of retinal images using eye gaze analysis
ANOVA	Analysis of variance
AOI	Areas of interest
AT	Assistive technology
B	Blue
BCI	Brain–computer interface
BeGaze	Behavioral and Gaze Analysis
BU	Bottom-up
CHT	Circle Hough transform
CR	Concentration ratio
CT	Computed tomography
CVA	Computational visual attention
DC	Direct current
DIARETDB0	Diabetic Retinopathy Database
DPI	Dual Purkinje Image
DRIVE	Digital Retinal Images for Vessel Extraction
DRIONS-DB	Digital Retinal Images for Optic Nerve Segmentation database
Du	Duration threshold

EEG	Electroencephalogram
EGODD	Eye gaze–based optic disc detection
EGDPA	Eye gaze data processing and analysis
EOG	Electrooculography
FASD	Fetal alcohol spectrum disorders
FCM	Fuzzy c-means
FETDKB	Feature extraction and top-down knowledge building
FIS	Fuzzy inference system
FIT	Feature Integration Theory
FOV	Field of view
FOA	Focus of attention
FSD	Filter–subtract–decimate
G	Green
GUI	Graphical user interface
I-DT	Dispersion-threshold fixation identification
IG	Information gain
I-VT	Velocity-threshold fixation identification
INSPIRE	Iowa Normative Set for Processing Images of the REtina
HP	Hewlett-Packard
MM	Mathematical Morphology
IK	Itti–Koch
KL	Kullback–Leibler
MR	Magnetic resonance
MESSIDOR	Methods to Evaluate Segmentation and Indexing Techniques in the Field of Retinal Ophthalmology
ms	Millisecond

OD	Optic disc
ONH	Optic nerve head
ONHSD	Optic Nerve Head Segmentation Dataset
PCA	Principal component analysis
PD	Parkinson's disease
PET	Positron emission tomography
R	Red
ROI	Region of interest
RGB	Red, green, blue
STARE	STructured Analysis of REtina
SBGFRLS	Selective Binary and Gaussian Filtering Regularized Level Set
SVM	Support vector machines
TP	True positive
TD	Top-down
TIFF	Tag image file format
USB	Universal serial bus
UX	User experience
VAODD	Visual attention–based optic disc detection
VR	Virtual reality
WI	Wisconsin
WEKA	Waikato Environment for Knowledge Analysis
X-ray	X-radiation
^{0}	Visual angle
$\oplus$	Morphological dilation
$\ominus_e$	Morphological erosion

○	Morphological opening
•	Morphological closing
θ	Orientation angle
$\ominus$	Across scale difference
σ	Standard deviation

ABSTRACT

Eye movement includes the voluntary or involuntary movement of the eyes. The eye tracker device is used for measuring the eye movements. Eye gaze data analytics can bring out information about observer's age, sex, education, experience, visual processing, cognitive processing, and many more.

The thesis attempts to use the fact that the person's experience and expertise have an impact on their eye gaze pattern. The experts' eye gaze pattern while viewing the medical images depicts the attentional behaviour of the individual, which has been captured and further utilised for detecting the target region. The research work strives to automate and propose a complete eye gaze–based system that uses attentional theories inferred from eye gaze pattern.

The designed system is evaluated for detecting optic disc in fundus retinal image. The chosen topic has been interesting as optic disc detection is a fundamental task for retinal image processing for classifying other fundus structures and is crucial for the identification of eye-related diseases.

Owing to the fact that the human visual perception has been less studied for optic disc detection and an attempt to derive eye gaze based data analytics, the thesis first discovers how human perception works for optic disc detection using bottom-up visual attention model. The inference/ conclusions derived, paved way to propose an eye gaze–based optic disc detection (EGODD) system to detect optic disc in fundus retinal images. The eye gaze data while the user is performing simple target search task were collected from different users groups comprising of expert and nonexpert groups. Extensive data analysis has been carried to extract eye gaze features like fixation and using machine approach label regions in fundus retinal image. The segregated labelled data has been used to build a top down knowledge to bias the search map towards the target region.

The resulted Eye gaze based optic disc detection system (EGODD) was evaluated across standard fundus retinal datasets and compared against state-of-the-art methods. The EGODD system has been tested and validated for optic disc detection; nevertheless it can further be extended for other applications also.

CHAPTER 1

1 INTRODUCTION

1.1 Motivation

Eye tracking is a sensor-based technology that enables a device to know exactly where the eyes of a person are focused. It determines the presence, attention, focus, drowsiness, consciousness, or other mental states of the person. Eye tracking is the measurement of eye activity. Researchers make an attempt to address various questions, such as "Where do we look?" "What do we ignore?" "When do we blink?" and "How does the pupil react to different stimuli?" The answers to these questions if queried and interpreted become very complicated.

Eye-tracking field has been exciting field for researchers working across the globe on quite number of applications and areas. Researchers using eye tracking have achieved astonishing breakthrough (US20050105768A1, 2005; US9039419B2, 2015; US8774498B2, 2014 & WO2013150494A2, 2013). The eye-tracking research has wide applications in the field of automotive, medical, defense, industries, visual attention, advertising, entertainment, packaging, web design, and many more areas.

Within the preview of the research focus area of medical domain (Matsumoto et al. 2011; Bernal et al. 2014; Khan et al. 2012), it is observed that the eye-tracking research has been extensively applied to compare two groups, for example, experienced physicians and radiologists with the novice in the domain or comparison of patients with healthy controls. The research works reveals various theories associated to the behavioural difference between the two groups. It is found that domain experts' knowledge developed on the basis of their experience and education has an impact on the eye gaze pattern. This may be reason that eye tracking is used in training the novice in the domain using expert eye gaze data (U.S. Patent No. US9039419B2, 2015).

There are number of patented works that uses eye tracking for guiding user attention to important area in the image (U.S. Patent No. WO2013150494A2, 2013), for identifying the ignored regions (U.S. Patent No. US8311279B2, 2012), distracting regions (U.S. Patent No. US8929680B2, 2015) and for building a decision support system (U.S. Patent No. US20050105768A1, 2005). In most of these system eye tracker is important requirement for system to work (both for training and testing). The system which can work independent of eye tracker is essential in current age.

A parallel field visual attention looks at the interesting aspect of how humans look at images uses eye gaze data as a ground truth data to validate its hypothesis. The term "visual attention" refers to a set of cognitive operations that mediate the selection of relevant information and the filtering of irrelevant information from the environment/image. One of the unique qualities of the human vision system is that it quickly gains information regarding the environment and the objects in the environment using simple visual cues. The human visual attention systems are influenced by two main approaches namely, the bottom-up (BU) approach and the top-down (TD) approach. The BU approach is stimulus driven and consists of response to sudden changes that capture the attention in the image/environment. The top-down (TD) approach is a task-based action that is influenced by knowledge, goal, expectation, and emotion.

Various researches indicate that domain experts make use of their knowledge when they look at the images or videos in their field. It is a challenging task to develop a system that predicts, for specific target, where the domain experts/medical experts will look. Here, the aim of the research was to understand how target detection can be done by integrating the top-down (TD) approach along with bottom-up (BU) approach. This thesis describes the work that uses eye tracking for target detection, which attempts to detect the target region using the knowledge developed by domain experts' eye gaze pattern.

The optic disc (OD) detection is selected as target because of two reasons. First, the OD detection is an important and a necessary task for retinal image processing for identifying other fundus structures, such as macula and vessels. Second, the OD detection is essential to diagnose eye-related diseases, for example, hypertensive retinopathy, glaucoma, diabetic retinopathy, and hypertension.

So far, the investigation has been on how various image-processing techniques help us in detecting the OD region; however, human perception aspects are rarely investigated. The system here also considers human perception aspects in detecting the target region.

1.2   Scope of the Thesis

Immense potential is available in eye tracking technology. To bring this potential into solution is still a challenging task. An approach to study and infer the behavioural pattern while medical practitioner (expert) is viewing the medical images has been limited (Matsumoto et al. 2011; Bernal et al. 2014; Khan et al. 2012). Here, the observed inference has been modelled as a target detection system. The perspective is to provide a system which stays way ahead to build a knowledge base from the eye gaze data. The system can be deployed for variety of target detection application.

The thesis initially investigated on human perception behaviour while viewing an image stimulus for the search task application to detect target. The bottom-up (BU) visual attention model demonstrated the visual search behaviour of a user in terms of reaction time, pop-out theory, disjunctive and conjunctive search. The research attempts to incorporate domain experts' knowledge into the system. The way domain experts look at an image for a specific target is studied by using eye tracking. The system has also taken into account the features of the region that distracts attention from the target region. To understand the region that distracts attention from the target, eye gaze data from nonexpert group were collected. In this thesis, optic disc in the fundus retinal image is selected as the target. The domain experts are optometrists. The thesis then proposes an eye gaze–based target detection system based on the inference derived on the study on the expert eye gaze behaviour. The system is the integration of bottom-up (BU) and top-

3

down (TD) approaches. The system proposed here has been tested and validated using several standard fundus retinal datasets.

1.3 Objectives of the Thesis

The main objective of the thesis is to propose a novel prototype model, the Eye Gaze–based Optic Disc Detection (EGODD) system. The novelty of the system has been validated across research community, and a patent with specification no. 201641037789 and titled "System and method for detection of features in an image using knowledge of expert's eye gaze pattern" has been filed. The aim of the research work was:

- To investigate how bottom-up (BU) computational model works on fundus retinal images for OD detection.

- To investigate the behavioural difference between expert and nonexpert groups by studying their eye gaze patterns for the optic disc detection task.

- To develop a target detection system that integrates bottom-up (BU) and top-down (TD) approaches.

1.4 Contributions

In accordance with the objectives mentioned above the targeted research contributions will be the following:

- The visual attention based optic detection model was proposed which evaluates the search behaviour of the user while viewing disjunctive and conjunctive medical images. The need for top down knowledge to be integrated was proved with performance analysis of optic disc detection using bottom up approach.

- The behavioural difference between expert and nonexpert groups is investigated.

4

- An automated labelling system to distinguish target and non target regions from eye gaze behaviour of expert optometrists and nonexpert groups while viewing fundus retinal images has been developed.

- Proposed a novel target detection system that combines bottom-up (BU) and top-down (TD) approaches.

- The proposed system has been evaluated on multiple datasets and across various models for its performance.

1.5 Outline

The research work discussed in the thesis is organized into seven chapters. The literature survey is divided into two chapters. The basics of eye tracking and a critical review of the literature on eye gaze–based methods are given in Chapter 2. Chapter 3 introduces optic disc and gives a detailed literature survey on optic disc detection methods. It also highlights the identified research gaps.

In Chapter 4, the visual perception concepts are studied for optic disc detection using the bottom up visual attention system. The proposed visual attention–based optic disc detection (VAODD) approach is discussed in detail with analysing the effect of disjunctive and conjunctive search made on images. The performance of the system is validated with respect to standard dataset.

The Eye Gaze Based Optic Disc Detection (EGODD) system is proposed in Chapter 5. The experimental setup for eye gaze data collection, data processing, and eye gaze feature extraction is discussed. A comparison of the expert and nonexpert groups with statistical analysis illustrating the way experts and nonexperts looks at medical images.

In Chapter 6, the method for automatic labelling of attractor and distractor regions in fundus retinal images using eye gaze data is introduced.

In Chapter 7, the contribution of developing the top-down map to achieve the target has been modelled by using fuzzy based system. The results and evaluation of the eye gaze–based optic disc detection (EGODD) system are discussed with various performance metrics like success rate & overlapping score. The results of the eye gaze–based optic disc detection (EGODD) system are compared with the state-of-the-art OD detection methods to evaluate and prove its efficiency.

Finally, Chapter 8 presents thesis conclusions and highlights the contributions of the research work. It gives insight to the possible future direction the presented research can facilitate.

CHAPTER 2

2 LITERATURE SURVEY: EYE GAZE TRACKING

The research concentrates on the aspect of understanding the various areas where eye tracking is used. The focus of the research and the literature survey conducted here is on two major research areas: eye-tracking and optic disc detection. The basics of each research area are explained first, followed by a literature survey in that area.

This chapter focuses on eye-tracking area. The introduction to eye tracking is given in Section 2.1. The literature survey on eye tracking is explained in Section 2.2 followed by summary of the chapter in Section 2.3. The OD detection is discussed in Chapter 3.

2.1 Basics of Eye Tracking

Eye tracking is a sensor-based technology that enables the user of a device to know exactly where the eyes are focused. It ascertains one's presence, attention, focus, drowsiness, consciousness and other mental states. As shown in Figure 2.1, the observer's eye gazes are focused on the face of the boy, balloon, and banner.

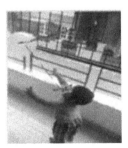

Figure 2.1 The observer's eye gazes focused on the face of the boy, balloon, and banner

2.1.1 Concept of Eye Tracking

Eye tracking commonly refers to the technique used to record and measure eye movements. It offers a new way of communicating with the human thought process. These eye movements indicate a person's gaze trajectory while performing a certain task. The *gaze* is the act of seeing and being seen. It is a steady intent look. Eye trackers are the devices that are used to measure the point of direction of the users' gaze, to identify the object on which the gaze falls.

Usually, the head position and the integration of eye are used to measure the location of the gaze in the visual scene. Simple eye trackers report only the direction of gaze relative to the head for a fixed position of the eyeball. Such eye-tracking systems are referred as intrusive systems because some special contacting devices are attached to the skin or eye to catch the user's gaze. The systems and the eye tracker apparatus that do not have any physical contact with the user are referred as nonintrusive systems or remote systems.

2.1.2 Eye-Tracking Technology

A number of eye gaze detection methods have been developed over the years. Direct visual observation of the eye gives a general indication of the character of eye movements (Yarbus, 1967). The experimenter could only observe large movements and could not notice the rotation of the eye through $1°$ and the corresponding movement of the eyes through 0.2 mm. Later, optical instruments such as lens, microscope, or specially devised instruments were used to detect small movements. Previously, several authors also used methods by which they established a mechanical connection between the eye and the recording system. The movement of the cornea was transmitted by three known methods: a lever and balance arm, an elastic balloon filled with air (eye movement-altered pressure), and attachment of a lever or thread to small cups (made of plaster of paris or aluminium). Low accuracy and a complicated setup meant that this method was outdated very quickly. Techniques mostly used in the twentieth century involve the use of electrooculography (EOG), scleral contact lens/search coil, and reflected light (limbus tracking, video-based combined pupil, and/or corneal reflection and dual Purkinje tracking). EOG relies on (DC signal) recordings of the electrical potential differences of the skin surrounding the ocular cavity. The changes can be detected using a pair of electrodes fixed to corresponding points of the skin and then amplified and recorded. The main advantage of this method is that it does not require a clear view of the eye, resulting in a large dynamic range. Techniques based on the corneal bright spot and still-and-motion-picture photography was also used in the early part of the twentieth century with relatively poor accuracy, as reported by Yarbus (1967). Methods used before the 1970s utilized invasive techniques that required tampering directly in the eyes. Such techniques, which are based on contact lens, offer high accuracy and large dynamic range but require an insertion into the eye. Mirror surfaces of the lens causing reflection of light beams or use of a search coil embedded in a scleral contact lens coil, which is then measured moving through an electromagnetic field (Vilariño et al., 2007), can be used to track eye positions.

The availability of image-processing hardware and possible applications of the gaze-tracking system for human–computer interaction prompted a revisit to the reflected light techniques due to their noninvasive nature. These tracking techniques use mainly infrared light to illuminate the eye, causing a reflection and/or sharper images of the eye. The sclera is a tough, opaque tissue that serves as the eye's protective outer coat. The iris is the coloured part of the eye. It controls light levels inside the eye similar to the aperture on a camera. The exterior of the iris, that is, the border between the iris and the sclera, is called the limbus. Limbus tracking requires optical detection of the boundary between the normally white sclera and darker iris. Occasional coverage of the top and bottom parts of the limbus by the eyelids is a limitation. A similar pupil-tracking method can also be used to observe the smaller and sharper boundary between the pupil and the iris. The shining of infrared light can also lead to several reflections on the boundaries of the lens and cornea (called **Purkinje** reflections). Four Purkinje reflections are created: two from the cornea and two from the lens (Figure 2.2). The first reflection (also called the **glint**) is measured relative to the location of

9

the pupil centre. This forms the basis of most current commercial eye-tracking systems.

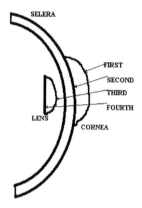

Figure 2.2 Purkinje Reflections

The DPI (Dual Purkinje Image) eye tracker (Robinson, 1963) tracks this first reflection along with the fourth to study gaze directions. It requires the head to be restricted and is relatively expensive. The weakness of the fourth reflection is that surrounding lighting must be heavily controlled. The video-based combined pupil and corneal reflection method uses these two ocular features to disambiguate head movement from eye rotation, and as a result does not need to have a fixed head unlike the DPI eye tracker.

2.1.3 The Eye and Its Movements

The human eye lets light in through the pupil, turns the image upside down in the lens, and projects it onto the back of the eyeball—the retina. The retina is filled with light-sensitive cells, called cones and rods that transduce the incoming light into electric signals sent through the optic nerve to the visual cortex for further processing. Cones are sensitive to what is known as high spatial frequency (also known as visual details) and provide us with colour vision. Rods are very sensitive to light and therefore support the vision under dim light condition.

There is a small area at the bottom of the eye, called the fovea (Figure 2.3). In this area, spanning less than 2° in the visual field, cones are extremely overrepresented. To see a selected object sharply, an individual therefore have to move his/her eyes, so that the light from the object falls directly on the fovea.

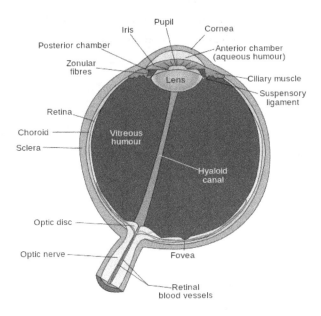

Figure 2.3 Anatomy of human eye (Rhcastilhos, 2007)

When the eye is still over a period of time, for example, when the eye temporarily stops at a word while reading, this is called a **fixation**, which lasts anywhere from some tens of milliseconds up to several seconds. **Fixation duration** shows the time in which eyes are relatively stable. The duration varies from 100 to 1000 ms, typically between 200 and 600 ms. The information from an image is almost entirely acquired during fixation.

The word *fixation* is a bit misleading because the eye is not completely still, but has three distinct types of micro-movements: tremor, microsaccades, and drifts. **Tremor** is a small movement of frequency, approximately 90 Hz, whose exact role is unclear. It can be imprecise muscle control. **Drifts** are slow movements taking the eye away from the centre of fixation, and the role of **microsaccades** is to quickly bring the eye back to its original position.

The rapid motion of the eye from one fixation to another is called **saccades**. Saccades are very fast typically taking 30–80 ms to complete. They rarely take the shortest path between two points, but can undergo one of the several shapes and curvatures. Duration of saccade is typically between 30 and 120 ms (Holmqvist et al., 2011).

If our eyes follow a bird across sky, we make a slower movement, called **smooth pursuit**. Saccade and smooth pursuit are completely different movements driven by different parts of the brain. Smooth pursuits require something to follow whereas saccades can be made on a white wall even in the dark, with no stimuli at all.

When a viewer focuses on an object for a longer duration, it is said to be an accurate perception and is considered to be a fixation. Thus, the maximum duration for every participant is recorded as a fixation point. The sequence of the eye movement is traced for a particular set of values for every individual and this is known as the scan path. **Blinks** are often identified as ($x = 0$, $y = 0$) coordinates or when pupil diameter is zero, indicative of a closed eyelid. Blink rate is defined as the number of blinks per second or minute (Holmqvist et al., 2011).

When the ROI is defined, one can count the **Dwell**. The dwell, often known as *gaze* in reading and *glance* in human factor, is defined as one visit in a region of interest (ROI), from entry to exit. **Dwell time** is defined as the sum of all fixation durations during a dwell in an ROI.

Pupil diameter is raw data provided as samples by the eye tracking device. The pupil diameter values are typically expressed in pixels of the eye camera. Some eye trackers can also report pupil diameter in millimetres after a calibration routine. Usually a horizontal pupil diameter is considered as a measure, because the vertical diameter is too sensitive to eyelid closure. This measure can be used to study a variety of cognitive and emotional states. The normal pupil size in adults varies from 2–4 mm in diameter in bright light to 4–8 mm in the dark (Holmqvist et al., 2011).

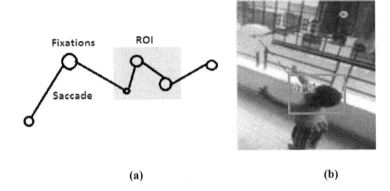

(a)   (b)

Figure 2.4 Representations of Fixations and Saccades

Figure 2.4(a) shows, six fixations. Three fixations are in the ROI, shown with the blue region. It has five saccades and one dwell. Similarly, Figure 2.4(b) has five fixations. Three in ROI shown with a red square. It has four saccades and one dwell.

The process of fixation identification is an important part of eye-movement data analysis. Three type of fixation detection algorithms are proposed in a study by Salvucci and Goldberg (2000). The categories are dispersion-based algorithm, velocity-based algorithm and area-based algorithm.

Dispersion-based algorithms are the most common types of detection algorithms. They have been most often used for low-speed data. Literature shows that it is the common choice for analysing 50-Hz data. Dispersion-based algorithms identify fixation by finding data samples that are close enough to one another for minimal time. They do not make use of velocity or acceleration information for calculation of fixations (Holmqvist et al., 2011). Dispersion-threshold identification (I-DT) proposed by Salvucci and Goldberg (2000) assumes that fixation points, due to their low velocity, are likely to cluster closely together. I-DT recognizes fixations as groups of consecutive points within a particular dispersion, or maximum separation.

Velocity-based algorithms focus on the velocity information in the eye-tracking data, assuming the fact that fixation points have low velocities and saccade points have high velocities. The velocity-based algorithm, velocity-threshold fixation identification (I-VT), described by Salvucci and Goldberg (2000), is the simplest of the identification methods that separate fixation and saccade points based on their point-to-point velocities. The velocity profiles of saccadic eye movements show essentially two distributions: low velocities for fixations (i.e., <100 deg/s) and high velocities (i.e., >300 deg/s) for saccades.

Area-based algorithms identify points within the given areas of interest (AOIs) that represent relevant visual targets (Salvucci & Goldberg, 2000).

The primary measurements used in eye-tracking research are fixations and saccades. There are also many derived metrics that arise from these basic measures, including gaze and scan path measurements. Pupil size and blink rate are also used by researchers. The commonly used eye movement metrics is given in Table 2.1 (Poole & Ball, 2005; Holmqvist et al., 2011).

Table 2.1 Commonly used eye movement metrics

Eye-Movement Metric	What it indicates
Number of fixations	More overall fixations indicate less efficient search (perhaps due to suboptimal layout of the interface).
Fixations per area of interest	More fixations on a particular area indicate that it is more noticeable, or more important, to the viewer than other areas.
Fixation duration	A longer fixation duration indicates the object is more engaging in some way, or some cases indicate difficulty in extracting information.
Number of saccades	More saccades indicate more searching.
Saccade amplitude	Larger saccades indicate more meaningful cues, as attention is drawn from a distance.
Regressive saccades (regressions)	Regressions indicate the presence of less meaningful cues.
Scan path duration	A longer-lasting scan path indicates less efficient scanning.
Number of dwells	It gives information about difficulty of a task.
Dwell time	Longer dwell time indicates informativeness of an object.
Pupil diameter	It gives information about mental workload, emotions, and drowsiness.
Blink rate	Blink rate increases with time on task and fatigue.

2.1.4 Types of Eye Trackers

Even if they all use same video-based pupil to corneal reflection measurement technology, eye trackers are very different among themselves. Basically, a video-based eye tracker has an infrared illumination and an eye-video camera, and typically an additional scene camera for a head-mounted eye tracker. Illumination(s) and eye camera(s) can be put on in front of the participants or on their head. Sometimes head tracking is added to the head-mounted system. Thus, this gives three types of eye tracker (Holmqvist et al., 2011).

The most common setup is the static eye tracker, which puts both illumination and eye camera on the table, in front of the participants. There are two subtypes— tower-mounted eye trackers and remote eye trackers, as shown in Figure 2.5(a). The tower-mounted eye trackers are in close contact with the participant whereas remote eye trackers are not at all or in very little contact with the participants, as shown in Figure 2.5(b).

The other common setup is the head-mounted eye tracker (Figure 2.5(c)), which puts both illumination and cameras on the head of the participant, mounted on a helmet, cap, or a pair of glasses.

The third type of setup adds a head tracker to the head-mounted eye tracker to calculate the position of the head in space.

The typical sampling rate of eye tracker systems ranges from 10 to 2000 Hz. The sampling frequency is measured in hertz (Hz). A 50 Hz eye tracker records the gaze direction of participants 50 times per second. More precise data can be collected with higher sampling frequency.

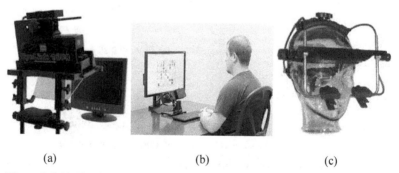

(a)   (b)   (c)

Figure 2.5 (a) The SR Research's EyeLink 1000 Tower Mount, (b) EyeLink 1000 Plus, and (c) EyeLink II eye trackers ("SR Research EyeLink," n.d.)

16

2.1.5 Manufacturers of Eye Trackers

The leading companies manufacturing eye trackers are SMI (SensoMotoric Instruments), Tobii, EyeLink, ISCAN, LC Technologies, EyeTech, The Eye Tribe (Although recently acquired by, and now owned by Oculus), Smart Eye, Mirametrix, Pupil Labs, Gazepoint, and Ergoneers ("Top 12 Eye Tracking Companies," 2017).

2.1.6 Applications of Eye Tracking

The eye-tracking methodologies mainly span neuroscience, psychology, industrial engineering, marketing, and computer science disciplines. For disabled users, an eye-tracking interface may be an indispensable form of communication (e.g., the eye is typing). The current and potential applications are summarized as follows:

1   Eye tracking serves as a viable alternative to conventional input devices (e.g., mouse and keyboard) for certain disabled users. This technology will continue to be useful for disabled users.

2   Eye tracking can potentially be used as a safety device or early warning system for indications of drowsiness or lack of concentration when operating machinery such as motor vehicles, power stations, and air traffic control systems.

3   Eye tracking is increasingly being used by marketing companies to investigate the usability of products and the effectiveness of advertisements. Analysing what potential customers may be looking for in an advertisement through objective data produced by an eye tracker can be used to optimize the effectiveness of the advertisements. Advertisements can take the form of TV commercials and printed and website advertisements.

4   Eye tracking serves as a good indication of interest for improving human–computer interaction. Eye-tracking interfaces can aid automatic scrolling function on screens, zooming interfaces, video conferencing, and so on. The improvement can vary from the system automatically issuing a command based on user's gaze behaviour to smart systems that can anticipate the user's need based on knowledge acquired by the system during real-time viewing.

However, outstanding issues (such as accuracy and interpretation) need further research.

5   Historically, eye tracking has been used for neurological and psychological research to understand the human visual system and its cognitive processes. Numerous findings have been useful for understanding certain neurological disorders and improving human–machine interaction with computer scientists.

6   Eye tracking can be used for applications that require visual inspections such as search and rescue operations, manufacturing defects, x-rays, and picture interpretation (art). Tracking eye movement of an expert visual inspection may be used to train novice inspectors providing a gaze pattern emerges.

2.2 Literature Survey on Eye Tracking

The study by Yang and Wang (2015) explores the recent development in using eye-tracking technology. The study has considered publication of 2354 articles during the years 1999 to November 2013. Countries with more than 10 articles are considered for the study. The study identified the five most prolific countries in eye-tracking research were USA (42.21%), UK (12.06%), Germany (11.72%), Canada (7.18%), and the Netherlands (6.58%). Scholars of the USA, the UK, Germany, Canada, and the Netherlands played important roles. Scholars in the countries with competences in eye-tracking technology have advantages in conducting eye-tracking research. This may be a reason why scholars in these countries contribute a significant proportion of eye-tracking articles (Yang & Wang, 2015).

As revealed by this study, there is very less contribution by eye-tracking researchers from India. There are many research fields where eye tracking is used. But it is seen from Figure 2.6 that more than half of the articles belong to the psychology-related fields (Yang & Wang, 2015).

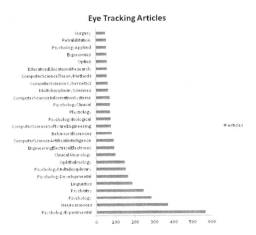

Figure 2.6 Distribution of eye-tracking articles by research fields. Data are taken from Yang and Wang (2015)

As discussed earlier, eye tracking has many applications. In the study here, application of eye tracking is restricted to assistive technology (AT), psychology and neuroscience, e-learning, and brain–computer interaction (BCT) and reading. This survey is carried to identify a broad range of applications covered by eye tacking. It is followed by a detailed discussion on application of eye tracking in medical domain.

Assistive technology (AT) is very helpful for people with disabilities. The technology helps them to accomplish tasks that they were unable to do (Balan et al., 2013). This will be especially helpful for most of neuro-disabled patients. Eye tracking and a computer can be used for word selection from a menu. The keywords are selected by the patient using eye-tracking technique (Lupu et al., 2012 & 2013). Such mobile devices are also helpful for people with restricted hand functions. It can be integrated in different VR and augmented reality systems for recovering and rehabilitation process targeting persons with neuromotor paralysis (Moldoveanu et al., 2013).

19

Roughly, eye motricity is a motor function of eye or, in simple term, related with the eye movements and is linked to the central nervous system. Thus, eye movements are strongly affected by disorders and diseases related to the cerebral cortex, the brainstem, or the cerebellum area. The study of eye movements can reveal the facts about which part of the brain is damaged and is a trusted indicator for dementia and a number of other brain-related diseases (Vidal et al., 2012). Eye movement information can also be used for health monitoring and assessment, for example, in autism, Alzheimer's disease, the acquired immunodeficiency syndrome dementia complex (AIDS dementia complex), multiple sclerosis, schizophrenia, and dyslexia (Lupu & Ungureanu, 2013).

In the e-learning, diverse technologies (e.g., collaborative software, cloud computing, virtual classroom) and dissimilar devices (e.g., mobile devices, webcams, audio/video systems) were used. The learner's behaviour can be studied using eye-tracking methods in e-learning. From eye tracking, it is possible to draw information about the user's level of attention, stress, relaxation, problem-solving, successfulness in learning, tiredness, interest level, focus of attention, or emotions. The level of motivation and interest in the learning system is observed using eye tracking (Al-Khalifa & George, 2010).

Brain–computer interface (BCI) is a direct communication pathway between the brain and an external electronic device, more often a computer. The BCI method in the study by Lee et al. (2010) combines BCI and eye tracking to analyse depth navigation, including selection and two-dimensional (2D) gaze direction.

The process of reading a word or a sentence becomes easy using eye tracking. The articles show how real-world reading can be investigated by eye-tracking and complementary methods, to understand how one reads, comprehends, and integrates texts in realistic, everyday scenarios (Jarodzka & Brand-Gruwel, 2017). The reports, which include text and pictures, describe how information given can be integrated with accompanying pictures to build a coherent mental model. Such works are increasingly being investigated with eye tracking over the past years (Mason et al., 2013; Jarodzka et al., 2015).

The VIP framework introduced by Ma et al. (2013) represents the eye gaze data as a function of visual stimulus, intent, and person. In the same line, the survey here tries to understand the for medical image stimulus, how persons' education, domain expertise affects their eye movements. In the successive paragraphs, a detailed discussion of eye gaze tracking for medical domain, specifically when two groups are involved, is presented. The survey was carried out to identify how the eye tracking is used to study behavioural differences of two groups. How eye tracking gives information about where a person is looking? Is there any difference in the way the domain experts will look to medical image than a novice in the domain?

The aim of the study conducted by Matsumoto et al. (2011) was to understand the areas of brain computed tomography (CT) images viewed by neurologists. The gaze distribution was compared with a saliency map to study the way in which attention is deployed by neurologists. The brain CT images showing cerebrovascular accidents were the stimulus, and twelve neurologists and twelve control subjects were the participants. The eye tracking device used was EyeLink 1000.

The heat map based on eye fixation and dwell time in ROIs was used to compare the two groups. The heat map shows the areas of images on which control subjects have more fixations are salient regions in the saliency map. The areas on which neurologists have often fixations were not always salient. Similar, the dwell time in neurologists was in clinically important area with low salience. Thus, it founds that neurologists purposefully look at clinically important areas when reading brain CT images. Here experts and control groups were compared. It was observed that both neurologists and control subjects used the BU salience form of visual attention, although the neurologists more effectively used the top-down instruction form.

The eye gaze patterns of the experts and novices were compared in Bernal et al. (2014). A study was conducted to identify visual search pattern differences between physicians with different levels of experience. Eye gaze data were recorded during the screening of colonoscopy videos for polyp search. Fixations were represented in the form of heat maps. The reaction time, dwelling time, and energy concentration ratio (CR) metrics were used for analysis. Experimental results show a significant difference between two groups and the obtained maps proved a helpful tool for characterization of the behaviour of each group.

A study of surgeons' eye movements was conducted by Law et al. (2004). The aim was to access surgeons' skills using their eye movements. The eye movements of five experts and five novices were compared. The task for the study was undertaken using a computer-based laparoscopic surgery simulator. As given, the experts were faster and committed fewer errors than novices. The results from the eye gaze analysis indicated that novices require more visual feedback of the tool position to complete the task than the expert. Similarly, experts sustained their eye gaze on the target while handling the tool whereas novices were more diverse in their behaviours.

A study on the eye gaze pattern of the novice and expert surgeons while watching surgical videos was conducted by Khan et al. (2012). The gaze patterns of expert surgeons and junior residents were analysed. The eye gaze data of expert surgeons were recorded when they were performing laparoscopic procedures in the operating room and when watching the operative video. Eye-gaze similarities in self-watching and others' watching were computed by the level of gaze overlay. There was 55% overlap and 43.8% overlap of the gaze reported. There was a notable difference reported between novice and expert surgeons.

The architecture given in Vilariño et al. (2007) includes video eye tracking for a set of specific issues, such us saliency identification, detection, and categorization of polyps in colonoscopy videos. In this work, the authors show how eye tracking can provide reliable and massive datasets in an efficient way. The gaze position data can provide useful information for the identification of the salient traits to which the experts are focusing their attention during the polyp identification process. The authors showed that the datasets obtained by eye tracking can be used to train powerful classifiers, such as a support vector machine (SVM).

An approach for designing radiology workstations is given by Atkins et al. (2006). They have designed a look-alike radiology task with artificial stimuli. The task involved a comparative visual search of two side-by-side images, using two interaction techniques. The eye gaze data from the four radiologists was collected while they performed the task. The duration of the fixations on the controls, the left and right images, and on the artificial targets was measured. Here the results show that disruption of visual search leads to cognitive disruption; subjects use the left image as a reference image and multiple saccades between left and right side images are necessary because of the limitations of the visual working memory. This article shows that computer interaction techniques can be analysed by using eye gaze data. This eye gaze data are also helpful to find search strategies.

A method was devised by Tseng et al. (2012) where participants watched television while their eye movements were recorded. The eye-tracking data from patients and controls were combined with a computational model of visual attention to extract features. The results showed that with eye movement traces recorded from 15 min of videos, they classified Parkinson's disease (PD) versus age-matched controls with 89.6% accuracy (probability 63.2%), and attention-deficit hyperactivity disorder (ADHD) versus foetal alcohol spectrum disorder (FASD) versus control children with 77.3% accuracy (probability 40.4%). Here the eye gaze data were used for classifying patient and healthy control. All these methods are summarized in Table 2.2.

23

Table 2.2 Literature survey on eye gaze tracking in medical domain

Authors	Tasks	Eye-Tracking-Related Metric	Participants	Inferences	Statistical Analysis
Matsumoto et al. (2011)	View brain computed tomography images	Fixations, heat map	12 neurologists and 12 control subjects	It is found that neurologists use their experience while looking at the images	Statistical analysis was performed using ANOVA
Bernal et al. (2014)	Polyp search	Number of fixations, duration of the fixations, dwelling time	22 physicians	Most of the expert fixations were on the target	Statistical analysis was performed by sign test, and Wilcoxon signed-rank test
Law et al. (2004)	Computer-based laparoscopic surgery simulator	Gaze time on the tool gaze accuracy	Five experts and Five novice surgeons	Experts found more efficient for the task as compared with novice	Statistical analysis was performed by ANOVA
Khan et al. (2012)	Performing laparoscopic procedures in the operating room	Level of gaze overlay	Two expert surgeons and junior residents surgeons	Difference between gaze pattern between two groups was identified	Statistical analysis was performed by ANOVA
Atkins et al. (2006)	Visual search on artificial stimuli	Duration of the fixations, number of fixations on regions of interest	Four radiologists	Eye gaze tracking shows that disruption of visual search leads to cognitive disruption	–
Tseng et al. (2012)	Watch video	Oculomotor, group and saliency-based features	21 ADHD, 31 FASD, 14 PD 18, and 24 controls	It is observed that eye gaze patterns of the healthy and patient were different	Statistical analysis was performed by ANOVA

The literature survey shows that the eye tracking in medical domain usually aims for comparison and target search. Matsumoto et al. (2011) compared expert neurologists and control while they were viewing the brain CT images. Bernal et al. (2014) compared the expert and novice physicians for target as polyp search. Khan et al. (2012) compared the eye gaze pattern of the novice and expert surgeons while they were watching surgical videos. Tseng et al. (2012) used eye gaze features for classification of patients and controls. The methods here target on classifying and comparing the participants. Vilariño et al. (2007) used eye tracking for target, that is, polyp in colonoscopy videos detection.

Thus, it becomes clear that all the works were carried out to compare and to conclude on the behaviour difference of two groups. The investigation is needed to further use these differences in different aspects. It is observed from the survey that the domain experts' experience has great influence on the identified regions. The research is required to understand how the domain experts' experience can be used for a building system.

Along with the research papers, the patents that use eye tracking are also surveyed. This survey was carried out to identify how eye tracking is applied for various applications.

The system with U.S. Patent No. US20050105768A1 (2005) aims for manipulation of image data by extracting attributes of a set of image using eye-tracking technique, to construct a decision support system. A method in this patent comprises carrying out eye tracking on an observer observing the image and applying factor analysis to the fixation regions to identify the underlying image attributes that the observer is seeking. The fixate region of image has been identified by an observer by analysing fixation points and saccadic eye movements. The information on fixation points is fed to feature extraction library. Explicit domain knowledge is used to identify relevant image attributes.

The skill acquisition interface is given in U.S. Patent No. US9039419B2 (2015), which discusses a method for training novices. This invention supports transfer of skills from expert to novice. A method and system for capturing expert behaviour, such as gaze patterns, is discussed here and a catalogue (e.g., database) of these behaviours is created. In this patent, gaze patterns of the two groups are compared. When there is a deviation of novice gaze pattern from stored expert gaze pattern, the correction is made by creating movements of image, colour change of the image, or intensity change in the image to help promotion of novice behaviour to expert level. It compares in real time the behaviour of second users with stored first user.

The method for detection and identification of anomalies in target images, with respect to reference images, is given in U.S. Patent No. WO2013150494A2 (2013). It aims for visual exploration of an image during target search. Using a user's attention distribution, it produces a feedback. This feedback gives the user an indication of the efficacy of the exploration. The system here guides the user's attention toward the parts of the image deemed important and not yet adequately explored by the user by superimposing dynamic markers on the image. The system also aims to suggest optimal scan path to the user, that is, best image exploration strategy. Main processing includes two expert systems. The first expert system establishes a series of points of the image deemed to be relevant as a function of a specific predefined target. It organizes points in the form of relevance matrix. The second expert system collects eye gaze data from the user and processes the data. The fixations are categorized based on a threshold and relevance matrix.

The method given in U.S. Patent No. US8774498B2 (2014) extracts features representative of patches of the image to generate weighting factors for the features based on location relevance data. The weighting factors are then used to form a representation of the image.

The method given in U.S. Patent No. US8929680B2 (2015) discloses a visual attention map to represent one or more regions of an image. A salient region map defines one or more regions of the image as salient. An intersection between the visual attention map and the salient region map is determined to identify a distracting element in the image. Here, the attention map and a salient region map can be calculated using eye tracking.

The ignored region identification method is given in U.S. Patent No. US8311279B2 (2012). It tracks gaze data of the first user and collects initial gaze data, which include a plurality of gaze points, for the first user. The system identifies one or more ignored regions of the image based on a distribution of the gaze data within the image and displays subset of the image. The subset of the image is selected so as to include an ignored region of the one or more ignored regions and is displayed in a manner that draws attention to the respective ignored region.

The invention, U.S. Patent No. US8824779B1 (2014), exemplified as a single-lens stereo optics design with a stepped mirror system for tracking the eye, isolates landmark features in the separate images and locates the pupil in the eye. It matches landmarks to a template centred on the pupil, mathematically traces refracted rays back from the matched image points through the cornea to the inner structure, and locates these structures from the intersection of the rays for the separate stereo views.

The methods for assessing and/or diagnosing neurobehavioural disorder in a subject are given in U.S. Patent No. US20100208205A1 (2010). In this method, the participant was freely viewing a visual scene. A computational model was used to select one or more features in a visual scene and generate a spatial map having first map values that were predictive of eye movement endpoints of a hypothetical observer relative to the one or more features. A difference between second map values corresponding to the subject's eye movement endpoints and a set of map values selected randomly from the first map values was quantified, wherein the difference was indicative of a neurobehavioural disorder in the subject. These patents are summarized in Table 2.3.

An attempt was made in U.S. Patent No. US9039419B2 (2015) to train the novice in the domain using experts gaze behaviour using eye tracking. It compared the behaviour of a user with that of the stored expert user in real time. The eye tracking was also used for guiding the user's attention (U.S. Patent No. WO2013150494A2, 2013). It involved a single user. The image data manipulation was carried out by extracting set of image attributes using eye-tracking technique to construct the decision support system (U.S. Patent No. US20050105768A1, 2005). The ignored regions were identified with the eye-tracking technique (U.S. Patent No. US8311279B2, 2012). The distracting element in an image was identified in U.S. Patent No. US8929680B2 (2015).

In most cases, one or two participants were involved. Most of the systems had eye tracker as an essential element required for the system to work. Nevertheless, to deploy an automated system, eye tracker is a crucial and costly requirement. The system design that can work independent of the hardware is a vital need of the current era.

Table 2.3 Patents related to eye tracking

Patents	Year	Title	Novelty
US20050105768A1	2005	Manipulation of image data	To construct a decision support system. To understand which image attribute contributes to observer performance
US9039419B2	2015	Method and system for controlling skill acquisition interfaces	To control skill acquisition interface. To provide a method for training the novices
WO2013150494A2	2013	Method and system for improving the visual exploration of an image during a target search	To improve visual exploration of an image during target search. To guide the user's attention toward the parts of the image deemed important
US8774498B2	2014	Modelling images as sets of weighted features	To extract features representative of patches of the image To form a representation of the image
US8929680B2	2015	Method, apparatus, and system for identifying distracting elements in an image	To identify where the user is distracted
US8311279 B2	2012	System and method for improved image analysis through gaze data feedback	To identify ignored regions in the image
US 20100208205 A1	2010	Eye-tracking method and system for screening human diseases	To assess and/or diagnose a neurobehavioural disorder in a participant

2.3 Summary

The chapter highlights the immense amount of work done in the field of eye tracking. The eye tracker device is used to measure eye movements. There has been finite number of eye tracker available from various manufactures. Most popular eye trackers are remote eye tracker and head-mounted eye tracker.

Different eye movements, such as fixation, saccades, scan path, and blinks, have been discussed in this chapter. Compared with the other eye movements, fixation carries most of the information. Well-known fixation detection algorithms have been explored in the chapter.

According to the literature survey, most of the eye-tracking research is carried out in the countries such as the USA, UK, Germany, Canada, and the Netherlands. The statistics of eye tracking research shows that eye tracking research in India is meagre.

A survey was carried out to identify how eye tracking is applied for different applications such as AT, psychology and neuroscience, e-learning and BCI, and reading. The focus was on the applications of eye tracking in medical domain. The patents also surveyed to understand applicability of eye tracking for different problems. For various applications, eye tracking played a crucial role. The following chapter focuses on basics of OD and literature survey in OD detection field.

CHAPTER 3

3 LITERATURE SURVEY: OPTIC DISC DETECTION*

Medical imaging is the technique and process of creating visual representations of the interior of a body for clinical analysis and medical intervention, as well as visual representation of the function of some organs or tissues. There are various types of medical images, for example, X-ray images, radiography images, magnetic resonance images, medical ultrasonography or ultrasound images, fundus retinal images, endoscopy images, elastography images, brain CT images, and positron emission tomography images. The medical images are examined by the experts to identify anatomical structures, to monitor changes by comparing sequential images, and to plan for better treatment. In clinical ophthalmology, colour retinal fundus images acquired from digital fundus camera are widely used to detect and diagnose eye-related diseases. The automatic detection of landmark anatomical structures, optic disc (OD), macular region, and retinal blood vessels is needed for detecting and diagnosing diseases. Thus, the interest of the ophthalmologists is to locate these anatomical structures.

One of the important parts of the anatomical structures of human eye is the OD. The OD detection is essential in ophthalmic image processing. This is the main step in classifying other fundus structures (macular region and retinal blood vessels).

----

* A part of this chapter has been published as, "A study on current optic disc detection methods," in *Proceedings of 2nd International Conference on Sustainable Computing Techniques in Engineering, Science and Management* and in *International Journal of Control Theory and Applications*, 2016, Volume 9, Issue 40, pp. 441–452.

31

Light received by the human eye is transmitted to the brain through the optic nerve. The OD is the point of exit for ganglion cell axons leaving the eye.

Because of the absence of rods or cones, the OD corresponds to a small physiological blind spot in each eye. In a normal human eye, the OD carries 1–1.2 million neurons from the eye to the brain. The OD is oval shaped, brighter than surrounding, and about 2 mm in diameter (Figure 3.1).

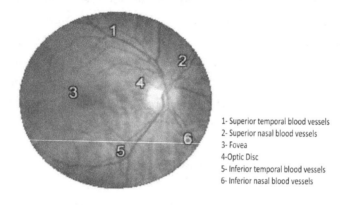

1- Superior temporal blood vessels
2- Superior nasal blood vessels
3- Fovea
4- Optic Disc
5- Inferior temporal blood vessels
6- Inferior nasal blood vessels

Figure 3.1 Retinal components of the human eye (Osareh, 2004)

The change in shape and size of OD results in ophthalmic diseases such as glaucoma, diabetic retinopathy, and hypertension. These diseases result in visual impairment in the early stage and blindness in the later stages. In a few cases, these problems are due to ageing, obesity, and so on. Early diagnosis and proper treatment are needed to avoid visual impairment and blindness ("Prevention of blindness and visual impairment," 2009). Because OD detection is a crucial requirement in the retinal image processing, the focus of this research is on OD detection. The chapter discusses the fundamental concepts of OD and state-of-the-art methods used for OD detection.

The OD basics are explained in Section 3.1. Techniques used for OD detection are given in Section 3.2 and literature survey on OD detection methods is given in

Section 3.3. Identified research gaps are discussed in Section 3.4 followed by the summary of the chapter in Section 3.5.

3.1 Basics of Optic Disc

In fundus retinal image, OD has a bright yellowish colour with a whitish central cupping; from this cupping the central retinal artery and vein pass. This section discusses about the fundus photography and publicly available datasets.

3.1.1 Fundus Photography

Fundus, Latin for the word "bottom," is an anatomical term referring to the portion of an organ opposite from its opening. Fundus of eye is the back portion of the interior of the eyeball, visible through the pupil by use of the ophthalmoscope. In fundus photography, fundus cameras with an intricate microscope are used. The OD, central and peripheral retina, and macula are structures that can be visualized on a fundus photo ("Ophthalmic Photographers' Society," n.d.). The bright yellow region in Figure 3.1 is the OD or optic nerve head (ONH). From the centre of the optic nerve radiates the major blood vessels of the retina. Approximately 4.5–5 mm to the left of the disc can be seen a slightly oval-shaped, blood vessel-free spot, the fovea, which is at the centre of the area known as the macula by ophthalmologists. A circular field of approximately 6 mm around the fovea is considered the central retina while beyond this is peripheral retina, 21 mm from the centre of the retina (fovea). The total retina is a circular disc of between 30 and 40 mm in diameter (Kolb, 2011).

3.1.2 Publicly Available Fundus Retinal Image Datasets

Most of the retinal OD segmentation methodologies are tested on various publicly available datasets, for example, the DRIVE, STARE, MESSIDOR, and INSPIRE datasets. Many OD detection methods use local dataset along with the standard fundus datasets available. In this section, a brief summary of the standard retinal datasets available is provided.

DRIVE Dataset: The Digital Retinal Images for Vessel Extraction (DRIVE) dataset (Staal et al., 2004) consists of 40 colour fundus images.

STARE Dataset: The STructured Analysis of the REtina (STARE) dataset (Hoover et al., 2000) is funded by the US National Institutes of Health. The project has 400 fundus images.

MESSIDOR Dataset: The MESSIDOR dataset (Decencière et al., 2014) contains 1200 images in two sets; the images were captured in three ophthalmological departments by a research program sponsored by the French Ministries of Research and Defense.

DIARETDB0 Dataset: The Standard Diabetic Retinopathy Database Calibration level 0 DIARETDB0 (Kauppi et al., 2006) comprises 130 colour fundus images, 20 normal, and 110 with signs of diabetic retinopathy, acquired from the Kuopio University Hospital in Finland.

DIARETDB1 Dataset: The diabetic retinopathy database and evaluation protocol DIARETDB1 (Kauppi et al., 2007) consists of 89 colour fundus images acquired from the Kuopio University Hospital in Finland. The dataset consists of 84 images with diabetic retinopathy and 4 normal images.

INSPIRE Dataset: INSPIRE stands for Iowa Normative Set for Processing Images of the REtina (Niemeijer et al., 2011). INSPIRE-AVR consists of 40 colour images of the vessels and OD and an arteriovenous ratio reference standard.

DRIONS-DB: Digital Retinal Images for Optic Nerve Segmentation Database (Carmona et al., 2008) is a public database for benchmarking ONH segmentation of digital retinal images. The database consists of 110 colour digital retinal images belonging to the Ophthalmology Service at Miguel Servet Hospital, Saragossa (Spain).

ONHSD Dataset: This dataset contains 99 fundus images taken from 50 patients randomly sampled from a diabetic retinopathy screening program; 96 images have discernible ONH (Lowell et al., 2004). A summary of the datasets discussed is provided in Table 3.1.

Table 3.1 Summary of fundus retinal image datasets

Dataset Name	Camera Used	FOA (Field of View)	No. of Images	Country
DRIVE	Canon CR5 non-mydriatic 3CCD	45°	40	Netherlands
STARE	Topcon TRV-50	35°	400	USA
MESSIDOR	Topcon TRC NW6 3CCD	45°	1200	France
DIARETDB0	Digital fundus camera	50°	130	Finland
DIARETDB0	Digital fundus camera	50°	89	Finland
INSPIRE	-	-	40	USA
DRIONS-DB	Colour analogical fundus camera	-	110	Spain
ONHSD	Canon CR6 45 MNf fundus camera	45°	99	UK

3.2 Techniques Used for Optic Disc Detection

The OD detection methods available in the literature can be broadly classified into image processing–based methods (Wisaeng et al., 2014; Khalid et al., 2014; Muntasa et al., 2015; Mithun et al., 2014; Dehghani et al., 2012; Fraga et al., 2012; Tjandrasa et al., 2012; Godse & Bormane, 2013; Welfer et al., 2013; Kande et al., 2008; Sopharak et al., 2008; Wang et al., 2015) and visual attention–based method (Gutte & Vaidya, 2014). In this section, the basic introduction to commonly used image-processing techniques for OD detection and visual attention is given followed by the state-of-the-art OD detection.

3.2.1 Image-Processing Basics

Image processing is a method used to convert an image into digital form and to perform some operations on it, to get an enhanced image or to extract some useful information from it. It is a type of signal dispensation in which input is image, such as video frame or photograph, and output may be image or characteristics associated with that image. There are many image-processing techniques used for OD detection. In this section, most commonly used image-processing techniques for OD detection are discussed.

Mathematical Morphology (MM) is considered as the science of appearance, shape, and organization (Jayaraman et al., 2009). It is most commonly applied to digital images. It is also the base of morphological image processing, which consists of a set of operators that transform images. MM was originally developed for binary images and was later expanded to grayscale functions and images. In digital image processing, MM deals with nonlinear processes that can be applied to an image to remove details smaller than a certain reference shape, usually called the structuring element.

The most common morphological operations used in image processing are dilation, erosion, opening, and closing. **Dilation** is an operation in which the binary image is expanded from its original shape. The amount of expansion is controlled by the structuring element. If X is the reference image and B the structuring element, the dilation of $X \times B$ is represented as:

$$X \oplus B = \{Z | [(\hat{A})z \cap X] \subseteq X\} \qquad (3.1)$$

where $\hat{A}$ is the image B rotated about the origin. When an image X is dilated by a structuring element B, the outcome element Z would be that there will be at least one element in B that intersects with an element in X.

Erosion is a thinning operation that shrinks an image. The extent by which shrinking takes place is determined by the structuring element. Here, if there is a complete overlapping with the structuring element, the pixel is set white or 0. The erosion of X by B is given as:

$$X \ominus_e B = \{Z | [(B)z] \subseteq X\} \qquad (3.2)$$

In erosion, the outcome element Z is considered only when the structuring element is a subset or equal to the binary image X.

Opening operation is performed by first doing an erosion, followed by a dilation. Opening smoothens the inside of object contours, breaks narrow strips, and eliminates thin portions of the image. It is mathematically represented as:

$$X \circ B = (X \ominus_e B) \oplus B \qquad (3.3)$$

Closing operation does the opposite of opening. It is dilation followed by erosion. Closing fills small gaps and holes in a single-pixel object. The closing process is represented by:

$$X \bullet B = (X \oplus B) \ominus_e B \qquad (3.4)$$

Closing operation protects coarse structures, closes small gaps, and rounds off concave corners.

Circular Hough Transform (CHT) is a basic technique used in digital image processing for detecting circular objects in a digital image. CHT is a specialization of Hough transform. The purpose of the technique is to find circles in imperfect image inputs. The circle candidates are produced by "voting" in the Hough parameter space and then selecting the local maxima in a so-called accumulator matrix.

Image Histogram is a graphical representation of the lightness/colour distribution in a digital image. It plots the number of pixels for each value. It is a spatial domain technique. Histogram of an image represents relative frequency of occurrence of various grey levels. The histogram of a digital image with grey levels in the range $[0, L - 1]$ is a discrete function:

$$h(r_k) = n_k \qquad (3.5)$$

where r_k is the kth grey level and n_k is the number of pixels in the image having gray level r_k. Histogram of images provides a global description of their appearance.

Image segmentation is the process of partitioning a digital image into multiple segments. The segmentation aims to simplify and/or change the representation of an image into something that is more relevant and easier to analyse. Image segmentation is commonly used to detect objects and boundaries (lines, curves, etc.) in images. In the segmentation process, labels are assigned to every pixel in an image such that pixels with the same label share certain characteristics. The easiest method of image segmentation is called the thresholding method, which is based on a threshold value to convert a grayscale image into a binary image. Several popular methods are used in industry including the maximum entropy method, Otsu's method (maximum variance), and k-means clustering.

The Otsu's algorithm assumes that the image contains two classes of pixels following bi-modal histogram (foreground and background pixels); it then calculates the optimum threshold separating the two classes so that their combined spread (intra-class variance) is minimal, or equivalent (because the sum of pair-wise squared distances is constant), so that their interclass variance is maximal. The Otsu's method exhaustively searched for the threshold that minimizes the intra-class variance (the variance within the class), defined as a weighted sum of variances of the two classes [Equation (3.6)]:

$$\sigma_w^2(t) = w_0(t)\sigma_0^2(t) + w_1(t)\sigma_1^2(t) \tag{3.6}$$

where weights w_0 and w_1 are the probabilities of the two classes separated by a threshold t and σ_0^2 and σ_1^2 are variances of these two classes.

Edge detection is a well-known image-processing technique. Region boundaries and edges are closely associated, because there is often a sharp adjustment in intensity at the region horizons. Hence edge detection techniques have been used along with segmentation techniques.

3.2.2 Visual Attention Basics

Saliency intuitively indicates some parts of a scene. These could be objects or regions that appear to an observer predominantly relative to their neighbouring parts. The area of the image attended visually is deemed as salient. The term *salient* is often considered in the context of bottom-up (BU) calculations (Itti & Koch, 2001; Koch & Ullman, 1985). Computational visual attention (CVA) is an artificial intelligence technique for simulating this biometric mechanism. With this mechanism, the difference in feature between region centre and surround would be emphasized and integrated in a conspicuity map.

Attention is the cognitive process of selectively concentrating on a discrete aspect of information while neglecting other information. Visual attention is the process of selectively attending to an area of the visual field while ignoring the surrounding visual areas. It is a common notion covering all factors that impact selection mechanisms, whether they are scene-driven BU or expectation-driven TD. It is a process in human perception that selects relevant regions from a scene and provides the regions for higher-level processing as object recognition. This makes it possible for us to act effectively in our environment despite the complexity of perceivable sensor data. The basis of many attention models dates back to "**Feature Integration Theory (FIT)**" put forth by Treisman and Gelade (1980). In this study, the author stated which visual features are valuable and how they are connected to direct human attention over pop-out and conjunction search tasks. The theory states that there are two stages of visual processing. In the first stage, called a pre-attentive stage, certain features in visual field are processed rapidly and without one's knowledge, for example, object's colour, shape, lines, textures, and curves. Two brain areas are involved in visual processing. The first area deals with colour, lines, textures, and so on whereas the second area deals with movements. In the second stage, all the features of the objects in the scene are recombined into whole object. The objects that are highly different from its vicinity stand out. The experiment conducted by Treisman and Gelade shows that prior knowledge helps a person to use attention effectively for feature combination.

Koch and Ullman (1985) put forth a feed-forward model to combine these features and proposed the concept of a saliency map, which is a topographic map representing conspicuousness of scene locations. The authors also proposed a winner-take-all neural network that selects the most salient locations and uses an inhibition of return mechanism to allow the user to shift the focus of attention to the next most salient location. Although FIT (Treisman & Gelade, 1980) explains the saliency of different locations of a visual input, what makes these locations salient is partially addressed by visual search paradigms. A task of active scan in the visual field for a particular object is called visual search.

Visual Search is everyday human activity. Looking for a known person in a busy place is an common example. It is also vital in diagnosing diseases as radiologists' search for lesions and other abnormalities in medical images before issuing reports. Searching salient regions in an image has also been of interest in computer vision because visually important features in an image are generally invariant to many image transformations and carry important image information (Elazary & Itti, 2008). There are two major types of search: one **is disjunctive search or feature search**, and the other is **conjunction search** as introduced by Treisman and Gelade (1980). In a search when the target and distractors are completely different, it is called disjunctive search. They are different by properties such as shape, colour, size, or orientation. For example, a red circle located within a group of green circles, as shown in Figure 3.2(a). The disjunctive types of search gives fast and correct responses most of the time. It is known as pop-out effect. When the target and distractors share more than one property, a serial attention is required to locate targets. Such type of search is called a conjunctive search. For example, if the target is red circles whereas distractors are made up of green circles and red squares, as shown in Figure 3.2(b). Therefore, the target shares colour but not shape with one type of distractors whereas target shares shape but not colour with another type of distractors. The common feature between target and distractors makes the search process difficult, resulting in a large search time. These cases are not having pop-out effect.

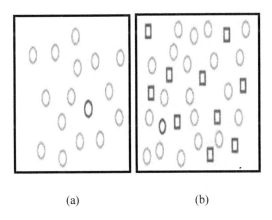

(a)   (b)

Figure 3.2 Sample stimulus showing (a) disjunctive and (b) conjunctive target searches

Feature Maps

In all psychological and computational models of attention the separate feature channels are used for processing of distinct features. In human brain there are distinct neurons and separate brain areas dedicated for processing of certain features. But this process is more intertwined than implemented by most models. However, the distinction into many pathways for colour, motion, and depth coincides to some extent with the specific feature channels. Although these pathways may not present in their pure forms, they nevertheless refer to the bias of certain brain regions. Three of the suggested neural pathways generally coincide each with one psychological feature channel, namely motion, colour, and depth, whereas there are several psychological feature channels for processing (Frintrop, 2006).

Centre-Surround Mechanisms

The centre-surround mechanism identifies feature contrast regarding intensity or colour. It is used in many computational and psychological models of attention. These have their neuro-physiological correlation on many different places in the brain. Later, cells in the brain continue in responding to contrasts with these mechanisms (Frintrop, 2006).

Different spatial scales are created using Gaussian pyramids, which made of low pass filtering and sub sampling the input image continuously, for calculating the center surround difference. The gabor pyramids are used to obtain orientation maps. Most of the model uses Greenspan et al. (1994) method (Itti & Koch, 2001). Gabor filters are the product of a symmetric Gaussian with an oriented sinusoid and this stimulates the respective field structure of orientation-selective neurons in primary visual cortex.

Colour Perception

The perception and processing of colour starts in the retina with different types of photoreceptors. Three types of receptors have preferences for red, green, and blue colours. Thereafter, the processing is continued from this trichromatic architecture to the opponent processing with the colour opponents red-green and blue-yellow. Usually, psychological models use a three-colour or double-opponency approach (Frintrop, 2006).

Saliency Map

Koch and Ullman (1985) propounded the idea of a saliency map to achieve pre-attentive selection, as given in Treisman (1988). This is a specific two-dimensional map that encodes the saliency of objects in the visual environment.

To compute the feature-specific saliency, the local values of the feature maps are compared to those of their surround. This operation is motivated from the on–off and off–on cells in the cortex and is also a general technique for detecting contrasts in images. The resulting contrasts were collected in so-called conspicuity maps, a term that has been since then frequently used to mean feature-dependent saliency (Frintrop, 2006).

3.3 Literature Survey on Optic Disc Detection Methods

The process for OD detection is commonly divided into four steps. The first is the pre-processing stage, which commonly aims to enhance the input image (e.g., contrast, sharpness, and illumination of the image; noise removal; and colour space conversion). These tasks are performed on the input image so as to make the image ready for processing. The second is the processing stage; here the process of isolating particular regions of interest (ROIs; OD here) within the image is carried out. The third is OD detection; here post-processing, for example, morphological operation, is performed, if required, to exactly detect OD. This step aims to describe and marking (i.e., annotating) either the external boundary or the internal skeleton of the objects/regions that are segmented in the fundus image. In the fourth step, analysis of the result is carried out by using performance measures.

3.3.1 Image-Processing Methods

The image-processing techniques for OD detection typically involve mathematical and morphological operations, Hough transform, histogram processing, segmentation, or thresholding.

The method described by Wisaeng et al. (2014) is depicted in the flowchart shown in Figure 3.3. Histogram specification is applied after normalizing the colour of the retinal images. The contrast enhancement is carried out between the OD and the retina background to increase the likelihood of OD detection. A median filtering operation is applied to the intensity band. Finally, original retinal image (RGB space) is transformed in LUV colour space. After transformation, a morphology method and Otsu's algorithms are applied.

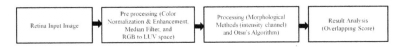

Figure 3.3 Flowchart for algorithm by Wisaeng et al. (2014)

The morphological closing operation is applied to the intensity channel of grayscale image. This is required to eliminate blood vessels and to create a constant OD region. The global image is thresholded using Otsu's method. The result of retinal image is binarized with thresholding. The result reported is with

91.35% accuracy for the STARE dataset and with an accuracy of 97.61% for the local dataset.

Sopharak et al. (2008) used morphological methods to detect the OD in retinal images. They do not discuss their method performance for the correct OD localization. Welfer et al. (2013) provided an adaptive morphological method for the automatic detection of the OD in digital colour eye fundus images. This method was able to detect the OD centre with 100% accuracy for the DRIVE database and with 97.75% accuracy for DIARETDB1 database. The colour morphology in Lab space to have a homogeneous OD region was used by Kande et al. (2008). The boundary of the OD is located using geometric active contours with variational formulation. The method by Mithun et al. (2014) automatically detected OD and blood vessel of retinal image, as shown in Figure 3.4. Pre-processing is carried out by global thresholding. First, OD is detected from blue plane of image using global thresholding, feature extraction, and morphological operation. A global threshold is determined by using Otsu method (Otsu, 1979). For a normal image, most of the bright pixels stay inside OD. Morphological operations are used to obtain the complete OD region. The features used for extraction include area, the ratio of the major and minor axes, and the length of the major and minor axes.

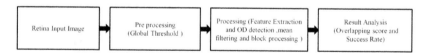

Figure 3.4 Flowchart for algorithm by Mithun et al. (2014)

Blob test is used to obtain these features. This subimage of OD is taken from the blue plane of the image. Small noises are removed using median filter. Then, the subimage is divided into smaller non-overlapping blocks and is analysed. The mean pixel area is calculated. The image is converted to black and white, with white in those regions that have area more than the mean and the other regions are converted into black. The bounding box is used for calculating centre and radius of the circle. Here, the DRIVE and STARE datasets are used. Performance is measured using the degree of overlap with the true OD. The calculated degree greater than 0.75 is considered to be successfully detected. For well-captured images, 100% success rate is reported.

Tjandrasa et al. (2012) applied the Hough transform as an initial level set for the active contours for OD segmentation, as shown in Figure 3.5. The OD segmentation steps start by converting the image to a grayscale image and then implementing the image preprocessing (image enhancement). Therefore, homomorphic filtering is applied to reduce the effect of uneven illumination. It has two stages: (1) applying a Gaussian low-pass filter, and (2) obtaining the filtered edge by performing dilation. The blood vessels are removed in the next step to facilitate the segmentation process. The threshold is applied to detect the low-pixel values in the image followed by applying the median filter to blur the blood vessels. Next, a circle that matched the location of OD is detected by performing a Hough transform. Subsequently, an active contour model is used to obtain the OD boundaries that are as close to the original OD boundaries as possible. The active contour model is applied with a special processing termed Selective Binary and Gaussian Filtering regularized Level Set (SBGFRLS) (Zhang et al., 2010). The algorithm achieved 75.56% accuracy using 30 images from the DRIVE dataset.

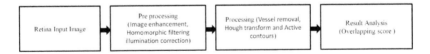

Figure 3.5 Flowchart for algorithm by Tjandrasa et al. (2012)

A hybrid method by Muntasa et al. (2015) for the OD detection in the retinal image is depicted in Figure 3.6. Blood vessels are filtered from retinal images using homomorphic and median filtering. Canny detection algorithm is used for edge detection because it is an optimal edge detection algorithm (Sheikh et al., 2015). To find circular shape in the image, the edge of the retinal image is extracted. OD detection is carried out using Hough transform. Forty retinal images from the INSPIRE dataset are used for the experiment in this research. This detection process reported 81.60% accuracy.

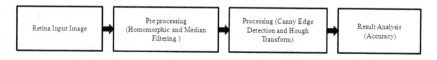

Figure 3.6 Flowchart for algorithm by Muntasa et al. (2015)

Akhade et al. (2014) used principal component analysis (PCA), MM, and CHT for OD detection. Flowchart is shown in Figure 3.7. Here the MESSIDOR database is used. Initially, RGB image is converted to a grayscale image. The PCA helps identify patterns in the data. These identified patterns then can be used to reduce its dimensions. In this method, three principal components of the fundus image are calculated. To remove blood vessels, MM operations are used. Closing operation is used for filling vassals. The circular patterns are detected using the CHT.

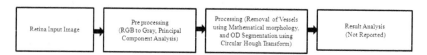

Figure 3.7 Flowchart for algorithm by Akhade et al. (2014)

Fraga et al. (2012) presented a methodology for the OD segmentation containing different stages, as shown in Figure 3.8. To decrease the contrast variability and increase the process reliability, the retinal image was normalized by the Retinex algorithm (Land & Mccann, 1971). Two different techniques were used to localize the OD: (1) analysing the convergence of the vessels (Hoover & Goldbaum, 2003) to detect the circular bright shapes, and (2) detecting the brightest circular area based on a fuzzy Hough transform (Blanco et al., 2006). After detecting the OD, the segmentation techniques were performed using the ROI specified by a difference in Gaussian filter. The vessel tree boundaries were segmented by Canny filter to compute the edges. The vessels' edges from the Canny output were suppressed using the vessel tree segmentation. Finally, the histogram information was included to measure the accuracy of segmentation. The methodology was evaluated on 120 images from the VARIA dataset. The method achieved 100% success rate of OD localization for both fuzzy convergence and Hough transform.

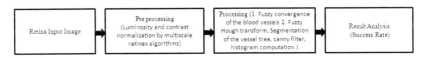

Figure 3.8 Flowchart for algorithm by Fraga et al. (2012)

Dehghani et al. (2012) provided a technique that used histogram matching for localizing the OD, as shown in Figure 3.9. Four retinal images from the DRIVE dataset were used to create three histograms from the colour image components (red, blue, and green) as a template. An average filter was applied to the image to reduce noise. The next step included extracting the OD for each retinal image using a window with a typical size of the OD. Then a template was created by obtaining a histogram for each colour component for each OD and by calculating the mean of the aforementioned histograms. To reduce the effect of pathological regions with high intensity, the histograms with intensity lower than 200 were used. The correlation between the histograms of each channel was calculated to gain the similarity of two histograms. Finally, thresholding was applied to the correlation function to localize the centre of the OD. The methodology was tested on three datasets: 40 images from the DRIVE dataset, 273 images from a local dataset, and 81 images from the STARE dataset, with the success rates being 100%, 98.9%, and 91.36%, respectively.

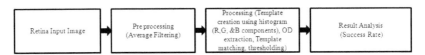

Figure 3.9 Flowchart for algorithm by Dehghani et al. (2012)

Aggarwal and Khare (2015) use a Kullback–Leibler (KL) divergence matching technique and vessel detection for OD detection in retinal images, as shown in Figure 3.10. OD is selected after reducing the effect of noise. This image is named as template image. For training 10 images were used. These template images were used to obtain the resultant image of OD. Histogram of these template images is calculated and then used for histogram matching. The histogram of green channel window was obtained. For histogram matching, KL divergence method was used (Khalid et al., 2005), which is a method used to calculate distance between template and moving histogram. This algorithm achieved 100% success rate for the DRIVE database and 90% success rate for the STARE database.

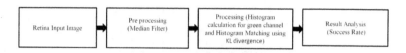

Figure 3.10 Flowchart for algorithm by Aggarwal and Khare (2015)

A flowchart of the system described by Godse and Bormane (2013) to locate an OD and its centre in retinal images is shown in Figure 3.11. Thresholding of green channel was used to find out candidate regions. Density criterion was applied to find out the OD region. The technique was developed and tested on standard databases provided for researchers on the Internet, DIARETDB0, DIARETDB1, DRIVE, and local databases. The local database images were collected from ophthalmic clinics. This system achieved 98.45% success rate to locate the OD and its centre for all tested cases.

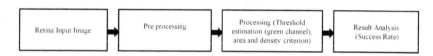

Figure 3.11 Flowchart for the algorithm by Godse and Bormane (2013)

Mendonça et al. (2013) used blood vessel network and intensity data to locate the OD, as shown in Figure 3.12. The distribution of vessel orientations around an image point was quantified using a new concept of entropy of vascular directions. This entropy was used to quantify both occurrence and diversity of vessel orientations around a pixel. After segmentation of the vascular network, a map with the entropy of vascular directions was prepared from the fundus image. An intensity map showing the Euclidean distance of the red (R) and green (G) components to origin of the RGB colour coordinates was also prepared from a colour image of the retina. The map was then segmented to retain just the pixels with the largest distance values, which were further analysed to generate a restricted set of high-intensity OD candidates. The initial OD location was the candidate where the maximum value of entropy occurred. Of the 1361 images of the four datasets, this method was able to obtain a valid location for the OD in 1357.

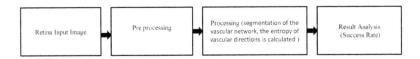

Figure 3.12 Flowchart for algorithm by Mendonça et al. (2013)

A method by Khalid et al. (2014) for OD and optic cup segmentation is shown in Figure 3.13. ROI (here OD and optic cup) cropping and colour channel analysis were carried out. Then, fundus images were used to determine the min, mean, and max values for the colour channel analysis. The fundus images were filtered using the green channel due to its better contrast than other colour channels. Dilation and erosion morphological operations were used to erase the blood vessel inside the OD and smoothen the intensity profiles around the centre of OD. Fuzzy C-Means (FCM) is used because of its accuracy in segmentation in the presence of intensity in homogeneities and because it can directly substitute into current methodologies that required hard segmentations, soft segmentations, gain field estimates, or in homogeneity-corrected images. Here the membership is assigned based on the distance between the cluster centre and the pixel. The closer the pixel to the cluster centre, the higher its membership.

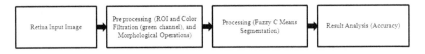

Figure 3.13 Flowchart for algorithm by Khalid et al. (2014)

The flowchart of the method by Lu and Lim (2011) is shown in Figure 3.14. This method used the unique circular brightness structure associated with the OD. The OD normally has a disc shape and is brighter than the surrounding pixels whose intensity becomes darker gradually with their distances from the OD centre. A line operator is used to identify such circular brightness structure. It also locates multiple line segments of specific orientations. The orientation and brightness variation were used to identify the OD region.

49

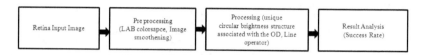

Figure 3.14 Flowchart for algorithm by Lu and Lim (2011)

Lupascu et al. (2008) proposed a method to determine the best circle that fits the OD. This method used texture descriptors and a regression-based method. The best circle was chosen from a set of circles determined with an innovative method, not using the Hough transform as past approaches. The method reported 95% success rate for the correct OD localization.

The template matching method was used by Wang et al. (2015) to approximately locate the OD, and the blood vessel was extracted to reset the centre. This was followed by applying the level set method, which incorporated edge term, distance-regularization term, and shape-prior term to segment the shape of the OD. The method reported success rate of 100%, 97.7%, and 97.75% for the DRIVE, DIARETDB0, and DIARETDB1 databases, respectively.

The use of approximate nearest neighbourhood for optic disc (OD) detection is discussed by Ramakanth and Babu (2014). In this approach, correspondence between the reference OD image and query image is identified. The correspondence helps to identify the closest match in query image with the reference image. OD was identified using the likelihood map that is calculated from distribution on patches in test image. The graph cut technique was used in Salazar-Gonzalez et al. (2014) for extraction of retina vascular structure. This vascular information is used to identify location of the OD. The prior intensity knowledge of the vessels along with the Markov random field image reconstruction method is used for detection of the OD. A dictionary-based method carried out in sparse representation framework is given in Sinha and Babu (2012). The dictionary of images which contains manually marked OD is created. The confidence map and blob detector is used to identify location of the OD in test image. The method is tested on DIARETDB0, DIARETDB1 and DRIVE datasets.

3.3.2 Visual Attention–Based Method

When there is an image or video specifically from the medical domain, then it is an interesting thing to study how humans will look or interpret such images. The visual attention system predicts human visual perception. An attempt was made by Gutte and Vaidya (2014). They used a BU visual attention model for salient object detection. The method starts with pre-processing of digital fundus images by contrast normalization throughout the image, and removal of blood vessels, which is major reason for distraction of finding OD candidate, using Bottom Hat Transform (Figure 3.15). Using this OD candidate, area of interest (AOI), that is, area surrounding OD and cup, is found. Then salient object detection algorithm is applied. The Itti's computational model for salient object detection is used. The method was tested on selected images from the MESSIDOR, STARE, and DRIVE datasets and from a local dataset. Of 529 images, OD was identified for 451 images, with success rate of 85.25%. The approach did not give an insight on the applicability of visual attention model for OD detection. The OD detection methods are summarized in Table 3.2.

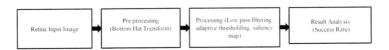

Figure 3.15 Flowchart for algorithm by Gutte and Vaidya (2014)

3.3.3 Deep Learning–Based Methods

In last five years, deep learning techniques have given new horizons in computer vision field. The deep retinal image understanding, a unified framework for vessel and OD segmentation, is given in Manini et al. (2016). The deep convolution neural network (CNN) is used for vessels and OD segmentation. Here, a CNN architecture that specialises a base network for the tasks of segmenting blood vessels and ODs in fundus images is designed. The DRIONS-DB and RIM-ONE (110 and 159 images, respectively) datasets were used for OD segmentation. The split of training and testing were (60/50 and 99/60, respectively).

Another deep learning approach proposed by Alghamdi et al. (2016) makes use of an end-to-end supervised model for OD abnormality detection. In this method, two successive learning-based models were used for identifying the OD and evaluating the abnormality.

A deep learning-based OD detection approach was presented by Lim et al. (2015). This method first identifies the OD region and exaggerates visual features from the region. A CNN is used to produce a pixel-level probability map. The map is used to predict disc and cup boundaries.

Table 3.2 Literature survey on optic disc detection techniques

Authors (Year)	Image-Processing Technique	Performance Metrics	Dataset and Number of Images	Result (%)
Wisaeng et al. (2014)	Morphology method (intensity channel) and Otsu's method	Average overlap	STARE 81 Local dataset 42	91.35 97.61
Sopharak et al. (2008)	Morphological methods	Success rate Average overlap	DRIVE DIARETDB1	95 and 59.55 16.88 and 29.41
Kande et al. (2008)	Colour morphology Geometric active contour	Success rate Average overlap	DRIVE DIARETDB1	95 and 86.51 29.66 and 33.41
Mithun et al. (2014)	Global thresholding (blue channel) Feature extraction and block processing	Success rate Average overlap	DRIVE 40 STARE 81	100 91.3
Tjandrasa et al. (2012)	Homomorphic filtering, Hough transform, and Active contours	Average overlap	DRIVE 30	75.56
Muntasa et al. (2015)	Homomorphic and Median filtering and Hough transform	Accuracy	INSPIRE 40	81.60
Akhade et al. (2014)	Mathematical morphology and circle Hough transform	-	MESSIDOR (subset)	-
Fraga et al. (2012)	Fuzzy convergence, Hough transform, and segmentation	Success rate	VARIA 120	100
Dehghani et al. (2012)	Histogram matching (red, green, and blue components), thresholding	Success rate	DRIVE 40 STARE 81 Local 237	100 91 98.9
Aggarwal and Khare (2015)	Median filtering, histogram calculation (green channel), and histogram matching	Success rate	DRIVE 40 STARE 20	100 90
Godse & Bormane (2013)	Thresholding (green channel), area estimation, and Hough transform	Success rate	DIRECTDB0, 1 DRIVE 40 and Local	98.45
Mendonça et al. (2013)	Entropy of vascular directions (red and green channels) and search for maximal values of entropy	Success rate	DRIVE 40 STARE 81 MESSIDOR 1200 INSPIRE 40	100 98.8 99.8 100
Khalid et al. (2014)	Colour filtering (green channel) Erosion and dilation with Fuzzy c-means (FCM)	Accuracy	High-resolution fundus images 27	93.7
Lu and Lim (2011)	Circular brightness structure and line operator	Success rate	DIARETDB0, 130 DIARETDB1, 89 DRIVE 40 STARE 81	97.4
Lupascu et al. (2008)	Texture descriptors and a regression-based method	Success rate Average overlap	DRIVE 40 DIARETDB1 89	95 and 88.76 40.01 and 30.95

(Continued)

Welfer et al. (2013)	Adaptive morphological method	Success rate Average overlap	DRIVE 40 DIARETDB1 89	100 and 97.75 42.54 and 44.58
Akyol et al. (2016)	Key point extraction, texture analysis, visual dictionary, and classifier techniques	Success rate	DIARETDB189 DRIVE 40 ROC 100	94.38 95 90
Wang et al. (2015)	Template matching Level set methods	Success rate Average overlap	DRIVE 40 DIARETDB0 130 DIARETDB1 89	100 , 97.7, and 97.75 88.7, 89.06 and 88.16
Ramakanth and Babu (2014)	Approximate Nearest Neighbour Field maps	Accuracy	DIARETDB0, DIARETDB1, DRIVE, STARE and MESSIDOR	99%
Sinha and Babu (2012)	Dictionary-based method, Blob detector	Accuracy	DIARETDB0, DIARETDB1 and DRIVE	97.6%
Gutte and Vaidya (2014)	Contrast normalization, Bottom Hat Transform, and bottom-up computational model	Success rate	MESIDOR, STARE, DRIVE, and local (selected images)	85.25

3.4 Research Gaps

The following research gaps were identified after surveying literature on eye tracking and optic disc detection.

A number of psychophysical and computational models of visual attention that take human visual perception into account have been suggested in the literature. Their main aim is to simulate the behavioural data and to better understand human perception. Most of these models have been studied and validated in the context of viewing natural scenes. The method by Gutte and Vaidya (2014) used saliency map to identify silent regions in the fundus image. It was tested only on selected images from the MESSIDOR, STARE, and DRIVE datasets and from a local dataset. There is need to study how BU computational model works for OD detection in fundus images. This is addressed in Chapter 4.

Most of the OD detection methods work on a specific image feature (e.g., colour and intensity). The method by Aggarwal and Khare (2014) used green channel of image. The method by Mithun et al. (2014) used blue channel and methods by

Godse and Bormane (2013) and Khalid et al. (2014) used green channel. Mendonça et al. (2013) used red and green channels of image. Dehghani et al. (2012) worked on red, green, and blue components of the image. Wisaeng et al. (2014) worked on intensity channel of image. The contribution made by different features for OD detection in fundus retinal images is need to study which is addressed in Chapter 7.

In majority of the target detection methods, learning mostly happens on the target region. There are certain regions in an image that distract attention. It is also important to have knowledge of the features of such distractors that distract attention from the target regions. The understanding of visual attributes that distinguish distractors from the target can improve search performance (Avraham et al., 2008). So, it is necessary to identify possible distractors in image which is discussed in Chapter 6.

It is observed that in eye tracking research when two groups are involved, the focus of the eye gaze research is on analysing the observer. The method by Matsumoto et al. (2011) compared expert neurologists and control while they were viewing the brain CT images. The method by Bernal et al. (2014) compared the expert and novice physicians for target such as polyp search. The eye gaze pattern of the novice and expert surgeons while watching surgical videos was compared by Khan et al. (2012). However, analysing the interaction between observer and the image needs to be investigated. The VIP framework introduced by Ma et al. (2013) captures the dependence of eye-gaze on Visual stimulus, Intent, and Person. In this research, for OD detection task, how the eye movements are affected by visual stimulus and person is investigated in Chapter 5 and 6.

By modelling the framework for OD detection, from the inference obtained from eye gaze data is represented as TD knowledge (This is discussed in Chapter 7).

3.5 Summary

The OD is an important element of the human eye. Detection of OD is necessary step for identifying different fundus structures and diagnosis of the diseases. The basic concepts, fundus photography, and standard datasets available for OD detection were discussed.

The extensive survey on the state-of-the-art research in the field of OD detection was carried out. The OD detection methods were classified into two categories: image processing based and visual attention based. It is observed that CHT, morphological operations, histograms processing, and thresholding were frequently used for OD detection.

The chapter summarises the importance of OD detection for diagnosis of the eye diseases. The discussion enlightens the existing research gaps in eye tracking and OD detection. The identified research gaps are used for problem formulation and have been further addressed in the upcoming chapters.

CHAPTER 4

4 VISUAL ATTENTION–BASED OPTIC DISC DETECTION[*]

The human visual perception is the ability of humans to interpret surrounding environment. When a person sees an image, there are certain areas in the image that attract attention. The computational visual attention (CVA) models try to predict the human visual perception behaviour. These models are based on the human visual perception concepts.

The literature survey reveals that currently there are many optic disc (OD) detection methods available. However, as discussed in the subsection 3.4, hardly there are any attention-based methods that perform OD detection. This chapter focuses on the applicability of CVA model for OD detection. In this chapter, the use of the bottom-up (BU) computational saliency model for fundus retinal images in the context of OD detection is investigated.

The BU computational saliency model identifies the salient regions in the images. The interest here is to understand whether the OD region in fundus images is considered the most salient region or not.

----

[*] A part of this chapter has been published as "Relevance of Computational Model for Detection of Optic Disc in Retinal images," in *International Journal of Computer Technology and Applications*, 2014, Volume 5-6, pp. 1896–1901.

The OD is an anatomical structure with a bright appearance. While identifying the OD region the major challenges are regions that share similar properties with the target. These regions are, for example, hard exudates (HEs), which are small white or yellowish white deposits, as shown in Figure 4.1. The HEs in a retinal image share similar characteristics with the OD.

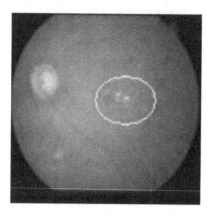

Figure 4.1 Sample retinal image showing yellowish white lesion (enclosed in white circle)

Thus, there is a need to categorize fundus images into two categories: with and without other regions sharing similar properties with OD. After consultation with the expert optometrists, the fundus images were classified into two types: disjunctive and conjunctive. Disjunctive images assume the target, that is, the OD, is the most salient region. On the other hand, conjunctive images assume other regions along with the target are salient.

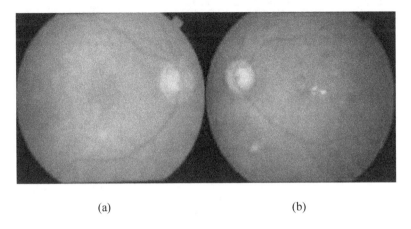

(a)   (b)

Figure 4.2 Retinal images showing (a) OD as disjunctive target and (b)
conjunctive target

Disjunctive types of fundus images are those that have the pop-out OD region. In
this case, the target region can be identified easily. Conjunctive types of fundus
images require focused attention. These images may have other regions that share
some similar properties with targets. Figure 4.2(a) shows disjunctive type of
image and Figure 4.2(b) shows conjunctive type of image.

The visual attention–based optic disc detection (VAODD) system is explained in
Section 4.1. Sections 4.2 and 4.3 describe, respectively, the results and summary
of this chapter.

4.1 Visual Attention–based Optic Disc Detection System

The major steps in the VAODD system are shown in Figure 4.3. The main dataset
used in this work is a subset of the STructured Analysis of the REtina (STARE)
project dataset (Hoover et al., 2000). The subset used contains 81 fundus retinal
images; 53 images are disjunctive type and 28 are conjunctive type. The Itti–Koch
(IK) (2001) computational BU saliency model is used for computation of saliency
map because it is a biologically motivated saliency model that closely follows
Feature Integration Theory (FIT) (Treisman & Gelade, 1980). As shown in Figure
4.3, the steps are divided into the following categories: pre-processing,
processing, and post processing.

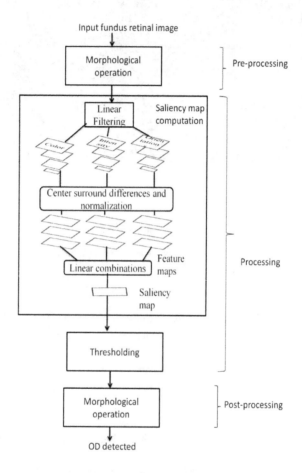

Figure 4.3 Major steps in the visual attention–based optic disc detection (VAODD) system

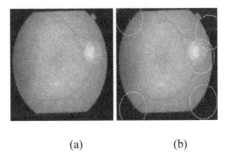

(a)   (b)

Figure 4.4 (a) Original image, (b) attended location by the IK model

4.1.1 Pre-processing

Usually, a wide variation is there in the colour, intensity, and orientation of the fundus retinal image foreground from background, as displayed in Figure 4.4(a). The identified locations using the IK model are displayed in Figure 4.4(b). The OD region is identified after attending all corners because of the presence of variation in colour, intensity, and orientation of the retinal image and its background.

Hence, a pre-processing step is required before using the IK model for computing saliency map for OD detection. The morphological opening operator ($\circ$) is applied to the original image (I_m) as pre-processing. The definition for the opening operation by structuring element B is given as follows:

$$Im_{pre} = \circ \ (B)(I_m) \tag{4.1}$$

where B is the disc-type morphological structuring element. The input image Im_{pre} is subtracted from the original image; the resulting image is used as input for processing.

4.1.2 Processing

In the processing step, saliency map is calculated using the IK model (Itti & Koch, 2001). First, the input image Im_{pre} is decomposed into a set of channels by using linear filters tuned to specific stimulus dimensions such as luminance, red, green, blue, and yellow hues or various local orientations. Such decomposition is performed at a number of spatial scales. This helps represent smaller and larger objects in separate subdivisions of these channels. Different spatial scales are created using Gaussian pyramids. Colour channels are created using the following equations:

$$Red = red - (green + blue)/2 \qquad (4.2)$$

$$Green = green - (red + blue)/2 \qquad (4.3)$$

$$Blue = blue - (red + green)/2 \qquad (4.4)$$

$$Yellow = red + green - 2(|red - green| + blue) \qquad (4.5)$$

$$Int = (red + green + blue)/3 \qquad (4.6)$$

Four Gaussian pyramids, Red (σ), Green (σ), Blue (σ), and Yellow (σ), are created from these colour channels. Int is use to create a Gaussian pyramid $Int(\sigma)$, where $\sigma \; \varepsilon \; [0..8]$. Local orientation information is obtained from Int using oriented Gabor pyramid O (σ, θ), where $\sigma \in [0..8]$ represents the scale and $\theta \in \{0°, 45°, 90°, 135°\}$ is the preferred orientation.

The centre-surround differences between a 'centre' fine scale c and a 'surround' coarser scale s give the feature maps, where $c \in \{2, 3, 4\}$ and $s = c + \delta, \delta \in \{3,4\}$. Each of the six red/green feature maps is created by first computing (red–green) at the centre, then subtracting (green–red) from the surround, and finally outputting the absolute value. Accordingly, maps $RG(c,s)$ are created in the IK model to simultaneously account for red/green and green/red double opponency [Equation (4.7)], and $BY(c,s)$ for blue/yellow and yellow/blue double opponency [Equation (4.8)]:

$$RG(c,s) = \left|\big(Red(c) - Green(c)\big) \ominus \big(Green(s) - Red(s)\big)\right| \qquad (4.7)$$

$$BY(c,s) = \left|\big(Blue(c) - Yellow(c)\big) \ominus \big(Yellow(s) - Blue(s)\big)\right| \qquad (4.8)$$

$$Int(c,s) = |Int(c) \ominus Int(s))| \qquad (4.9)$$

The orientation feature maps are obtained from absolute centre-surround differences between the orientation-selective channels. These maps, Ori (c, s, θ), encode, as a group, local orientation contrast between the centre and surround scales [Equation (4.10)]:

$$Ori(c, s, \ \theta) = \left|\left(Ori(c, \theta)\right) \ominus \left(Ori(s, \theta)\right)\right| \qquad (4.10)$$

In total, 42 feature maps are computed: 6 for intensity, 12 for colour, and 24 for orientation as given by Itti and Koch (2001). The conspicuity maps are created. The normalized maps are combined together to get the saliency map [Equation (4.11)]. The model gives most salient locations and outputs as saliency map.

$$Saliency\ Map \ = \ 1/3(\mathcal{N}\,(\overline{Int}) + \mathcal{N}\left(\overline{Color}\right) + \mathcal{N}\,(\overline{Ori})) \qquad (4.11)$$

To suppress the unwanted regions, binary segmentation is performed. A threshold, which is based on Otsu's algorithm, is used in thresholding. The purpose of thresholding is to change a grayscale image into a binary image, separating brighter regions from the dark background. The morphological open operation is applied on a binary image, which is then subtracted from the threshold binary image. I_{thresh} image is obtained after the thresholding of the saliency map. This image is further used for post processing.

4.1.3   Post processing

The morphological open operation ($\circ$) is used to remove small objects from an I_{thresh} image while preserving the shape and size of the larger objects in the image. As opening eliminates image details that are smaller than the structuring element used, it is easy to set the structuring element big enough to cover all likely vascular structures, but still small enough to preserve the actual edge of the OD:

$$I_{out} \ =\circ \ (B)(I_{thresh}) \qquad (4.12)$$

63

4.2 Result

The visual attention–based optic disc detection (VAODD) system is tested on 81 fundus images from the STARE dataset. The intermediate results of the VAODD system such as pre-processing, saliency map calculation, post processed image, and OD detection are shown in Figure 4.5. The fundus retinal image examples where the visual attention–based optic disc detection (VAODD) system fails to detect OD are shown in Figure 4.6. The result analysis is given in Table 4.1. It is able to detect OD in 43 of 53 disjunctive types of images and in 14 of 28 conjunctive types of images. For particular set of retinal images, it was found that the visual attention–based optic disc detection (VAODD) system takes average 6.36 s for disjunctive type of images and average 6.45 s for conjunctive type of images, as shown in Figure 4.7.

Table 4.1 Result analysis of the visual attention–based optic disc detection (VAODD) system

OD as Disjunctive Target 53 Images		OD as Conjunctive Target 28 Images		Total Images 81 Images	
Pass	Fail	Pass	Fail	Pass	Fail
46	7	14	14	60	21
Success Rate: 86.79%		Success Rate: 50%		Success Rate: 74.07%	

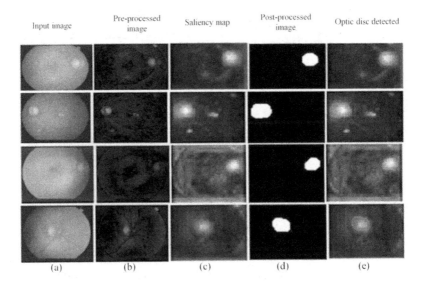

Figure 4.5 (a) Input retinal image, (b) result after pre-processing, (c) saliency map, (d) result after post processing, and (e) OD detected

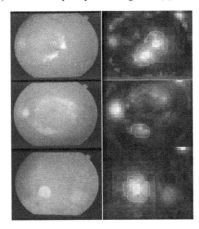

Figure 4.6 Examples where the visual attention–based optic disc detection (VAODD) system fails to detect the optic disc

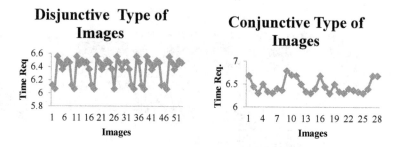

Figure 4.7 Time required by the proposed algorithm for both disjunctive and conjunctive cases (the time required is calculated after saliency map)

The analysis is carried out further to understand how BU approach in the IK model works for OD detection. After the computation of the saliency map, the maximum of the saliency map gives the most salient image location, to which the focus of attention (FOA) should be directed. It is observed that using the IK model for disjunctive type of images the FOA is one and for conjunctive types of images the FOA is varying, as shown in Figure 4.8. The example in which FOA is one and FOA is four on the fundus retinal image is shown in Figure 4.9.

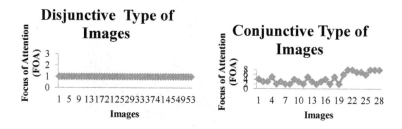

Figure 4.8 A saliency map that gives OD as pop up at first FOA (i.e., disjunctive case) (left) and OD as pop up at the successive FOA (i.e., conjunctive case) (right)

66

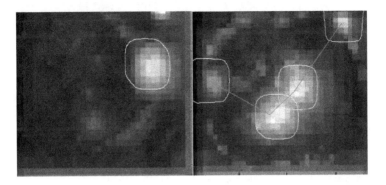

Figure 4.9 A saliency map that gives OD as pop up at first FOA on fundus image
(left) and OD as pop up at the fourth FOA on fundus image (right)

In this visual attention–based optic disc detection (VAODD) system work, the
role of the BU saliency model for OD detection on the STARE project dataset is
analysed. It is observed that for the images in which OD is a disjunctive type of
target, the success rate is 86.79% (47 out of 53 images) whereas images in which
OD is a conjunctive type of target, the success rate is 50% (14 out of 28 images).
The results show that the BU approach works well for the disjunctive type of
images, but the algorithm does not perform well for conjunctive type of images.
This indicates that BU approach is not enough for target detection. As the BU
saliency approach identifies all salient regions in images, so it may works for the
images where target is salient. Similarly, it is inferred from the experiment that
searching based on the knowledge of the target is not enough; knowledge of
distractors also plays an important role (Avraham et al., 2008; Nagy et al., 2005).

4.3 Summary

In this chapter, the relevance of the bottom-up (BU) saliency model in locating
OD in fundus retinal images is analysed. Results acquired show that the IK
saliency model with mathematical morphology and Otsu's algorithm functions
quite well in identifying OD in retinal images. The result shows 86.79% success
rate for images where OD is a disjunctive type of target and 50% success rate
where OD is a conjunctive type of target. It also shows that only the BU approach

is not enough for target detection. Knowledge of distractor regions along with the target regions may help improve the performance of the system. In Chapter 5, the eye gaze–based optic disc detection (EGODD) system is proposed, which combines the bottom-up (BU) and top-down (TD) approaches for OD detection.

CHAPTER 5

5 EYE GAZE–BASED OPTIC DISC DETECTION[*]

It is seen in Chapter 4 that the optic disc (OD) detection methods available in literature are mostly based on image-processing techniques. The human visual perception concepts are rarely considered for detecting OD. Similarly, it is observed that bottom-up (BU) approach alone does not perform efficiently for target detection applications.

Thus, the research here strives to propose a coherent system that combines BU and top-down (TD) approaches for target detection. The proposed eye gaze–based optic disc detection (EGODD) system is designed to identify the OD region automatically. It uses the knowledge developed from domain/medical experts' eye gaze pattern.

The eye gaze–based optic disc detection (EGODD) system tries to understand the possible regions in fundus images that can distract attention from the target region. The learning happens in the system based on the features of the target and distractor regions. The TD knowledge is implemented in the eye gaze–based optic disc detection (EGODD) system using the fuzzy system.

----

[*] A patent is filed on the eye gaze–based optic disc detection (EGODD) system discussed under **Specification No.** 201641037789 and **Patent Title** "SYSTEM AND METHOD FOR DETECTION OF FEATURES IN AN IMAGE USING KNOWLEDGE OF EXPERT'S EYE GAZE PATTERN."

*The paper on eye gaze–based optic disc detection (EGODD) system with title "Eye Gaze–Based Optic Disc Detection System." is published in Special Issue – Journal of Intelligent and Fuzzy Systems (SCI Impact Factor 2017: 1.261), 34 (2018) 1713–1722.

Here, the eye gaze–based optic disc detection (EGODD) system is evaluated for OD detection in fundus retinal images. Nevertheless, the system can be extended to different target detection applications as well.

This chapter introduces the eye gaze–based optic disc detection (EGODD) system. The system is organized into six units (Figure 5.1): the input unit, database, eye gaze data processing and analysis (EGDPA), automatic labelling of retinal images using eye gaze analysis (ALRIEGA), feature extraction and top-down knowledge building (FETDKB) unit, and test unit.

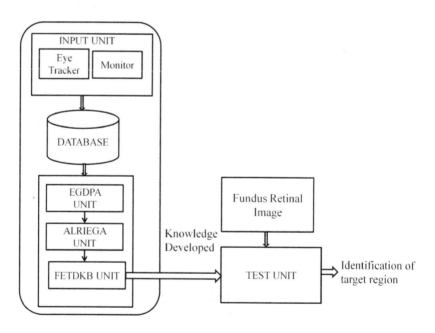

Figure 5.1 Block diagram of the eye gaze–based optic disc detection (EGODD) system

The graphical representation of the overall system is shown in Figure 5.2. Each unit is represented with a box. The input unit is designed to collect eye gaze data from two groups: one is expert optometrist group and the other is nonexpert group.

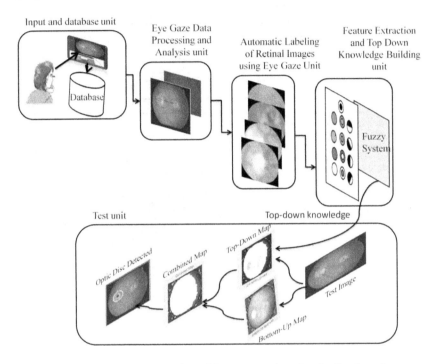

Figure 5.2 Graphical representation of the eye gaze–based optic disc detection (EGODD) system

71

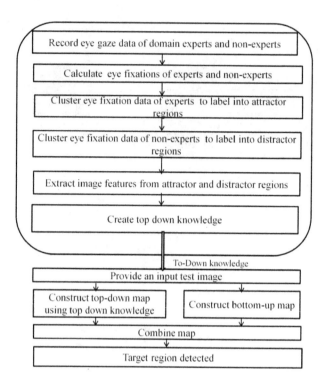

Figure 5.3 Major steps in the eye gaze–based optic disc detection (EGODD) system

The eye gaze data processing and analysis (EGDPA), automatic labelling of retinal images using eye gaze analysis (ALRIEGA), and feature extraction and top-down knowledge building (FETDKB) units deal with processing of eye gaze data, labelling of the regions, and feature extraction and top-down (TD) knowledge building, respectively. In the test unit, a fundus retinal image is given as input. Two maps, bottom-up (BU) and top-down (TD) maps, are generated. The combination of these maps gives the OD region. The input unit, Database, eye gaze data processing and analysis (EGDPA), automatic labelling of retinal images using eye gaze analysis (ALRIEGA), and feature extraction and top-down knowledge building (FETDKB) work offline. An eye tracker unit is required in the input unit where data collection takes place. Major steps in the eye gaze–based optic disc detection (EGODD) system are given in Figure 5.3.

The input and database units are explained in Section 5.1, the eye gaze data processing and analysis (EGDPA) unit is explained in Section 5.2, and the summary of the chapter is given in Section 5.3. The automatic labelling of retinal images using eye gaze analysis (ALRIEGA) unit is discussed in Chapter 6, and the feature extraction and top-down knowledge building (FETDKB) unit and test unit are discussed in Chapter 7.

5.1 Input and Database Units

The input unit consists of an eye tracker device and a laptop with stimulus image showing on laptop screen, as given in Figure 5.4.

The eye-tracking experiment is designed before actually starting the experiment. The experimental design includes participants, stimulus, and explanation of the experiment to the participants, and after participants agree for participation, actual experiment is conducted.

5.1.1 Participants

In this experiment, participants were selected from two categories. One category was of experts and the other one was of nonexperts. All participants had normal or corrected to normal vision. The experiment was conducted at the workplace for expert participants whereas for nonexperts, it was conducted in a university campus. The participants were tested individually. All the participants gave written consent to participate in the experiment. Initially, there were four expert optometrists (mean age 29.5 years) and ten nonexperts participants (engineering students and research scholars with mean age of 25.75 years).

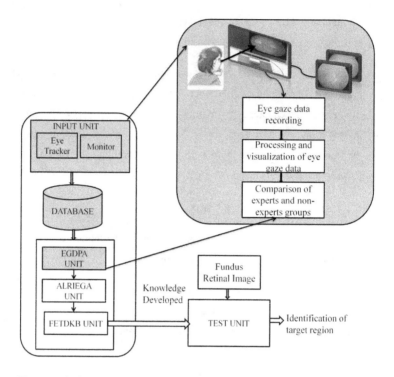

Figure 5.4 The eye gaze–based optic disc detection (EGODD) system with detailed view of input, database, and eye gaze data processing and analysis (EGDPA) unit

5.1.2 Stimulus Images

Eye gaze data were collected in two phases. In the first phase, a set of 25 fundus retinal images was selected as stimulus images for the experiment. Ten images were selected from the STARE dataset (Hoover et al., 2000) and fifteen images were selected from the DRIVE dataset (Staal et al., 2004). The set of stimulus images was termed as Dataset A.

In the second phase, a set of 95 images was used as stimulus images for eye gaze data collection. The 20 images were selected from the DIRECTDB 0 (Kauppi et al., 2006), High Resolution Fundus Images (Budai et al., 2013), and INSPIRE (Niemeijer et al., 2011). Twenty-five images were selected from the DRIVE and ten images were selected from the STARE. The set of stimulus images is termed

74

as Dataset B. After consultation with the expert optometrists, the fundus images were classified into two types: disjunctive and conjunctive. Disjunctive images assume the target, that is, the OD, is the most salient region. On the other hand, conjunctive images assume other regions along with the target are salient. Thus, the images are selected such as that final set contains both conjunctive and disjunctive type of images. The details about stimulus images selected for data collection are given in Table 5.1.

Table 5.1 Stimulus images selected from different standard databases

Datasets	Images Selected	Dataset
DRIVE	15	
STARE	10	**Dataset A**
DIRECTDB 0	20	
High Resolution Fundus Images	20	
INSPIRE	20	**Dataset B**
DRIVE	25	
STARE	10	

5.1.3 Hardware

The experiment was run on a Dell laptop, with screen size of 1366 cm × 768 cm, that was used to display stimulus images to the participants as well to collect eye-tracking data from them. The SMI iViewX RED-m (60 Hz; "SMI Eye Tracking," n.d.) eye tracker was fixed, as shown in Figure 5.5.

Participants faced the centre of the screen at a viewing distance of approximately 60–66 cm. They were instructed to restrict their head and body movements. The experiment was explained in detail to all participants.

5.1.4 Experimental Procedure

The experimental procedure followed for recording eye gaze is depicted in Figure 5.5. First, the experiment was explained to each participant, followed by taking their written consent for participation. The eye-tracking, calibration, and validation process were performed for each participant. The actual experiment was started after successful validation of the process.

75

The participants were instructed to look around the stimulus monitor and their eye movements were traced using SMI iViewX RED-m eye tracker. When a participant was sitting in an optimal position in front of the RED-m Eye tracking device, the eye-tracking monitor would show the user's eyes as two ovals somewhere near the centre. This means the user is at an ideal distance from the monitor and the eye-tracking device can track both the user's eyes. As shown in Figure 5.6(a), the user is sitting approximately 60 cm from the screen.

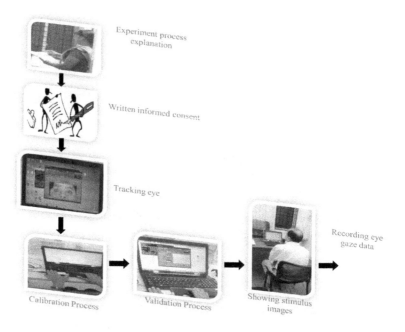

Figure 5.5 Experimental procedure

Calibration and Validation. The calibration and validation are important steps. In the calibration process, participants see a small circle on the screen, as shown in Figure 5.6(b). The participants were asked to follow the circle. Eye calibration requires participants to fixate on each point of a five-point grid displayed on the laptop screen.

76

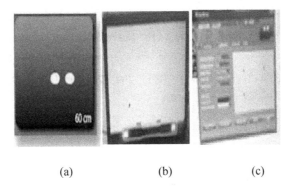

(a)   (b)   (c)

Figure 5.6 (a) Eye-tracking and viewing distance adjustment, (b) calibration, and (c) validation

To validate how well the calibration is immediately after calibration, the same procedure is repeated for validation. The red circle mark gives the validated points, as shown in Figure 5.6(c). If the calibration is good, the validated points will be closer to original points. The points that are farther indicate poor calibration, and in such case, the calibration process is repeated.

The stimulus images were shown in full-screen mode. All images were displayed sequentially one after another. The participants needed to watch the images and locate the target (i.e., OD). A program controlled the SMI iView X software and instructed it to record the movement of the participant's eye while watching the images. A total of 100 eye gaze samples from experts and 250 eye gaze samples from nonexperts were collected.

5.1.5 Database

The VIP framework given in Ma et al. (2013) shows dependence of eye-gaze on visual stimulus, intent, and person. It provides a common framework for eye gaze research. It represents the eye gaze data as a function of visual stimulus, intent, and person. Nonetheless, here the eye gaze data are represented as below.

EG, eye gaze data; m, number of sample/participants; n, number of stimulus images; $EG_{m,n}$, eye gaze data for participant number m and image number n

collected from two groups of participants. One is optometrists, called expert (E) here, and the other is nonexpert (NE), so $m \in \{E, NE\}$. The eye gaze data are in the form $EG_{m,n}$ (position X, position Y, duration), which is used for further processing. The eye gaze data collected from expert and nonexpert group were stored separately in a database.

5.2 Eye Gaze Data Processing and Analysis

As discussed in Chapter 2, the fixation is one of the main eye gaze features. There are two commonly used fixation detection algorithms: one is dispersion-based and the second is velocity-based algorithm. Fixations are mainly identified by a maximum allowed dispersion or velocity criterion. In dispersion-based algorithms (Salvucci & Goldberg, 2000), temporally adjacent samples must be located within a spatially limited region (typically 0.5–2.0°) for a minimum duration. In velocity-based algorithms, fixations are identified as contiguous portions of the gaze data where gaze velocity does not cross a predefined threshold (about 10–5°/s).

Typically, dispersion-based algorithms are used for data collected with a low-speed eye tracker. The velocity-based algorithms require data collected at the higher sampling rate (>200 Hz; Holmqvist et al., 2011). As the eye tracker device used for this research was having a sampling frequency of 60 Hz, so a dispersion-based algorithm was used in this study. This algorithm identifies fixations by finding data samples that are close enough to one another for a specified minimal period of time; for example, when the data samples are within 1° of visual angle at least for 150 ms, that sequence of data samples is considered as fixation (Figure 5.7). The pseudocode for fixation detection is based on Salvucci and Goldberg (2000) and is given in Figure 5.8.

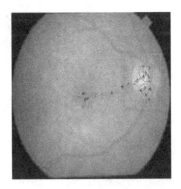

Figure 5.7 Representation of fixation: eye gaze data samples (red dots) must reside in green circle for a minimum amount of time to consider it as fixation

Input: ($EG_{m,n}$ (X, Y, Dur), dispersion threshold *dis*, duration threshold *du*)

Output: Fixation list

While there are still data samples

Step 1. Initialize window over the first sample to cover duration threshold *du*

Step 2. Calculate dispersion $d = \sqrt{(dx)^2 + (dy)^2}$

$$dx = \max(x_i) - \min(x_j)$$

$$dy = \max(y_i) - \min(y_j)$$

Step 3. While dispersion $d < dis$

Add data samples to the window.

Step 4. Note a fixation and duration. Add fixation point in file $EGFix_{m,n}$

Figure 5.8 Pseudocode for fixation detection

The algorithm will give a list of fixations in form $EGFix_{m,n}$(X_i position, Y_i position, duration$_i$). The fixations calculated for experts and nonexperts are shown in Figures 5.9(a) and (b), respectively.

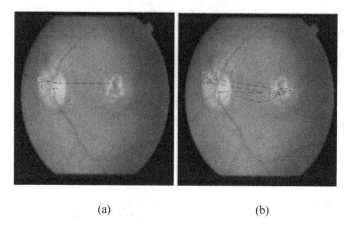

(a)   (b)

Figure 5.9 (a) Expert fixations, and (b) nonexpert fixations for fundus retinal image

The dispersion threshold (*dis*) can be set to 0.5°–1° of visual angle (Salvucci & Goldberg, 2000). The dispersion setting from 0.5° to 2° of visual angle is studied in Rotting (2001). The argument in the paper (Blignaut & Beelders, 2009) is that the optimal dispersion setting is 1°, but it relies heavily on the other parameters.

The duration threshold (*du*) can be set depending on task-processing demands. Rotting (2001) summarizes a number of studies that use dispersion algorithms and duration setting ranging from 60 to 120 ms. A 200 ms duration setting is used in Granka et al. (2008). The 200 ms setting has been commonly used in clinical studies, as given in Manor and Gordon (2003). The literature shows that duration threshold varies from 50 to 250 ms. In our research, dispersion threshold was set as 1° visual angle and the duration threshold was set as 150 ms.

The number of fixations, duration of fixation in ROI, number of dwells in ROI, dwell time in ROI, and the number of fixations in ROI for the expert and nonexpert groups were calculated. In this experiment, the OD region was the ROI. The graphs with different features are shown in Figure 5.10.

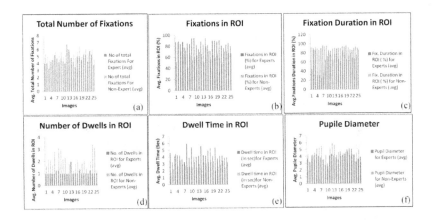

Figure 5.10 (a) Total number of fixations, (b) fixations in ROI, (c) fixation duration in ROI, (d) number of dwells in ROI, (e) dwell time in ROI, (f) pupil diameter

5.2.1 Visualization of Eye Gaze Fixations in Heat Map

Heat maps provide a quick, very intuitive, and in some cases, objective representation of eye-tracking data that naive users and even children can immediately grasp a meaning from. Their intuitiveness has made heat map visualizations very popular in parts of applied and scientific eye-tracking community. Their major advantage is that they very quickly give an easily digestible overview of the total data from a large number of participants. In the eye tracking for web usability field, heat map visualization is commonly used to describe the general outcome of an eye-tracking study (Holmqvist et al., 2011). For example, Nielsen (n.d.) refers to the well-quoted F-pattern: "Eye tracking visualization shows that users often read web pages in an F-shaped pattern: two horizontal strips followed by a vertical strip." Wulff (2007) uses heat maps to investigate how viewers explore web pages and concludes that only the very first links are looked at and the user does not read much on the page. Similarly, Bojko (2006) compares two page designs, using the heat map only to show that in one case, the gaze of the participants was focused only on the task-relevant target whereas in the other web page design, gaze was spread out (Holmqvist et al.,

2011). In this experiment, a heat map was developed to visualize where the experts and nonexperts look in fundus retinal images. The interest here is to know the eye movement behaviour of the two groups. The heat map was created from a set of discrete fixation points$(x_k, y_k), k \in [1, N]$, where N is the total number of fixation points found in an image and (x_k, y_k) is the location of the kth fixation point. Those fixation points are interpolated by a Gaussian function to generate a fixation density map $S(x, y)$, as given in Bernal et al. (2014):

$$S(x, y) = \frac{1}{N} \sum_{k=1}^{N} \frac{1}{2\pi\sigma_s^2} \exp \left(- \frac{(x - x_k)^2 + (y - y_k)^2}{2\sigma_s^2} \right) \tag{5.1}$$

where x and y denote, respectively, the horizontal and vertical positions of a pixel, and σ_s is the standard deviation of the Gaussian function. In this way, each fixation contributes to the heat map in a local neighbourhood centred in the fixation position and with an area of influence defined by σ_s. Therefore, in a region densely populated by fixations, a pixel has a brighter value than that in a more diffuse area. The σ_s is calculated by Equation (5.2), as suggested in Bernal et al. (2014).

$$\sigma_s = D * \tan \ (0.5\pi/180) \tag{5.2}$$

where D is the viewing distance between participant and display. The calculated heat map results are shown in Figure 5.11. The hot spots in the heat map point out the region that attracts participants' gaze. The expert's eye fixations were concentrated on the OD region compared with nonexpert's eye fixation. For example, Figure 5.11 shows the heat maps calculated from experts gaze are fully concentrated in the OD region whereas those calculated from nonexperts are comparatively scattered. The visualization of gaze plot, focus plot, scan path, and heat map for experts and nonexperts obtained using the Behavioural and Gaze Analysis (SMI BeGaze) is shown in Figure 5.12. BeGaze is the analysis program that comes with SMI eye trackers. It analyses data by structuring the information on experiments and subjects as well as showing the results as meaningful graphs.

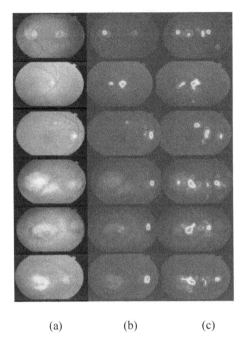

(a)   (b)   (c)

Figure 5.11 (a) Retinal image, (b) heat map of an average expert's fixation, (c) heat map of average nonexpert's fixations

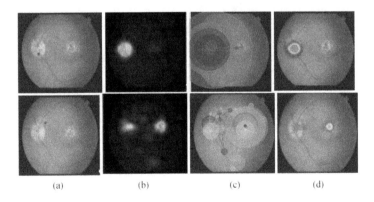

(a)   (b)   (c)   (d)

Figure 5.12 Visualization of fixation data: (a) gaze plot, (b) focus plot, (c) scan path, (d) heat map (upper row, expert's data; lower row, nonexpert's data) taken using BeGaze

5.2.2 Concentration Ratio

Concentration ratio (CR) is the percentage of the energy that falls under the OD. Here energy is calculated as the sum of heat map values. The formal definition of CR is given by Equation (5.3).

$$CR = 100 \times (E_{od}/E_t) \tag{5.3}$$

where E_{od} corresponds to the total energy under the OD and E_t corresponds to the total energy of the map for the whole image. A high CR value will correspond to a heat map focused on the OD whereas a low CR value will denote a more diffuse energy map (Bernal et al., 2014). As shown in Figure 5.13, for expert participants, CR value is higher compared to the nonexpert participants. It indicates that experts' focus is on the target OD whereas nonexperts' focus is attracted by other parts of the fundus image as well.

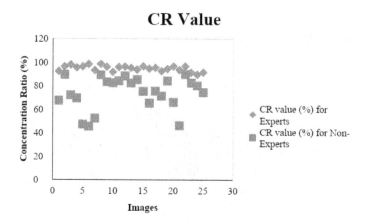

Figure 5.13 Scatter plot for concentration ratio of experts (avg.) and nonexperts (avg.)

5.2.3 Statistical Analysis

The statistical analysis was carried out for the expert and nonexpert group based on the number of fixations, pupil diameter, number of fixations in ROI, number of dwells, and dwell time in the ROI using one-way analysis of variance (ANOVA). The pseudocode for comparison of the expert and nonexpert groups is given in Figure 5.14. The mean and standard deviation for each feature are summarized in Table 5.2.

Input: Eye gaze features (total number of fixation, fixation in ROI, fixation duration in ROI, number of dwells in ROI, dwell time in ROI, pupil diameter) of the expert and nonexpert groups

Output: Statistical analysis of both groups

Step 1. For each feature, carry out a statistical analysis for both groups based on mean and variance

For mean, null, and alternative hypotheses

   H0: The means of two classes are equal.

   H1: The means of two classes are not equal.

For variance, null, and alternative hypotheses

   H0: The variances of two classes are equal.

   H1: The variances of the two classes are not equal.

Step 2. Calculate correlation between different features.

Step 3. Compare the expert group and nonexpert group based on the results of steps (a) and (b).

Figure 5.14 Pseudocode for comparing the expert and nonexpert groups

Table 5.2 Mean and standard deviation for expert and nonexpert groups

Features	Expert		Nonexpert	
	Mean	Std. Deviation	Mean	Std. Deviation
No. of fixations	4.66	0.80	5.02	0.50
No. of fixations in ROI (%)	85.11	6.05	61.08	16.09
Duration of fixation in ROI (%)	90.70	3.40	66.68	18.72
No. of dwells in ROI	1.08	0.21	1.97	0.68
Dwell time in ROI (s)	4.37	0.68	2.91	0.56
Pupil diameter	3.98	0.61	4.45	0.79

5.2.3.1   The Mean Test

The expert and nonexpert groups revealed differences in the mean test (Table 5.3): t critical two-tailed value is 2.0638.

Table 5.3 Mean test for the expert and nonexpert groups

Feature	t-Stat value
No. of fixations	−6.16
Number of fixations in ROI	8.48
Duration of fixation in ROI	6.22
No. of dwells in ROI	−6.24
Dwell time in ROI	7.65
Pupil diameter	−2.85

All above t-stat values lie in the critical region. So, the null hypothesis is rejected and the alternative hypothesis is accepted. The means of the two classes are not equal.

5.2.3.2   Variance Test

The variance test was performed between expert and nonexpert groups. The results are shown in Table 5.4.

Table 5.4 Variance test for the expert and nonexpert groups

Feature	Result
No. of fixations	$[F(1,48) = 11.992, p < 0.05]$
Number of fixations in ROI	$[F(1,48) = 70.996, p < 0.05]$
Duration of fixation in ROI	$[F(1,48) = 39.839, p < 0.05]$
No. of dwells in ROI	$[F(1,48) = 39.176, p < 0.05]$
Dwell time in ROI	$[F(1,48) = 67.515, p < 0.05]$
Pupil diameter	$[F(1,48) = 8.607, p < 0.05]$
Concentration ratio	$[F(1,48) = 55.13, p < 0.05]$

Large F values show that the null hypothesis should be rejected and the alternative hypothesis should be accepted. So the variances of the two classes are not equal. A significant difference was found between the two groups for all features. Collectively, result shows that expert and nonexpert groups behave differently for OD detection.

The inference from the analysis is as follows: experts were able to find target soon and fixate their gaze on the target; maximum experts gaze were concentrated on the target whereas nonexperts fixations were scattered throughout the image. After target identification, nonexperts found it less effective to fixate gaze on it. Experts' maximum fixations were in the OD region.

5.2.3.3   Correlation between Features

The correlation between eye gaze features for expert and nonexpert groups are as follows: a positive correlation was found between number of fixations in ROI and duration of fixation in ROI for experts $[r = 0.605, p = 0.001]$. A positive correlation was observed between number of fixations in ROI and dwell time in the ROI for experts with $[r = 0.416, p = 0.039]$. There is no correlation seen between the number of fixations and number of fixations in ROI, dwell time in the ROI, and number of dwells in ROI for the experts with $[r = 0.304$ and $r = -0.138, p > 0.05]$. Similarly, the number of fixations and number of fixations in ROI found to be independent for nonexperts with $[r = -0.394, p > 0.05]$. The number of fixations in the ROI and fixation duration in the ROI for nonexperts were not correlated with $[r = 0.241, p > 0.05]$. The number of fixations in the ROI and dwell time in the ROI, and dwell time in the ROI and number of dwells in the ROI were found to be independent with $[r = 0.139$ and $r = 0.118, p > 0.05]$. The scatter plots for all features for both groups are shown in Figure 5.15.

In the survey given in Jacob and Karn (2003), the number of fixations measure was found to be most common. In this experiment, results indicate that the experts have comparatively less total numbers of fixations. The fewer fixations may be because they avoid fixations on irrelevant parts of the image. This finding agrees with the literature. Rotting (2001) concludes that a low number of fixations could mean that the task goal has been reached, that the participant is experienced, or the search task is simple. The results showed that out of a total number of fixations by experts, the maximum fixations fall in the OD region, that is, the ROI.

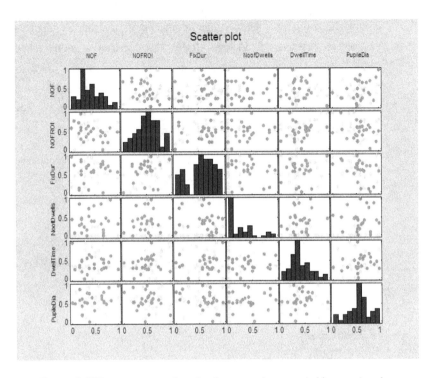

Figure 5.15 Feature scatter plots for the expert (represented in green) and nonexpert (represented in red) groups

Similarly, a high number of fixations for the nonexpert group may indicate difficulty in interpreting the fixated information, same as reported in Ehmke and Wilson (2007). It was also found from the results that the duration of the fixation in the ROI is higher for an expert. Longer fixation of the experts indicates that with increasing skill, more information is extracted around the point of fixation, making eye movements overall more efficient. A longer fixation duration is much connected with richer and more effortful cognitive processing (Henderson & Hollingworth, 1999). All these findings indicate a functional link between what is fixated and cognitive processing of that item—the longer the fixation, the deeper its processing (Holmqvist et al., 2011).

89

The higher dwell time indicates interest in an object or higher informativeness of an object (Friedman & Liebelt, 1981). This indicates a strong relationship between consecutive fixations on an item and how much one needs to mine information from it. It was observed that dwell time for an expert in the OD region was longer. The number of dwells in the ROI made by experts was comparatively less than that by the nonexperts.

There is no major difference in pupil diameter between expert and nonexperts, as revealed by the results. But it is observed that for disjunctive type of images, pupil diameter for both groups is closer whereas for conjunctive type of images, the pupil diameter of the nonexpert group is slightly larger. This may agree with the findings that mental workload increases the pupil diameter (Hess & Polt, 1964). CR is applied to estimate whether heat maps are concentrated on to OD or spread throughout the image. The comparability of the CR values indicates experts gazing on the OD when the image appears on the screen.

5.3 Summary

The eye gaze–based optic disc detection (EGODD) system, a combination of bottom-up (BU) and top-down (TD) approaches, has been introduced in this chapter. The block diagram, graphical representation, and the major steps involved in the system are discussed. The procedure for eye gaze data collection and processing is explained. Various eye gaze features such as fixation, fixation duration, and dwells were extracted from collected eye gaze data. The two groups, expert group and nonexpert group, were compared based on the extracted eye gaze features. It has been understood from the visualizations and statistical analyses that the expert and nonexpert groups behave differently for a given OD detection task. The gaze fixations of the expert group were concentrated on the OD region and those of the nonexpert groups were attracted by other regions of the fundus images as well. Chapter 6 discusses on how these differences are used for region labelling.

CHAPTER 6

6 REGION LABELLING OF RETINAL IMAGES USING EYE GAZE DATA *

In the specific field of research in medical domain, it is observed that the eye-tracking research has been extensively applied to compare two groups. The research works usually conclude on behavioural difference between the two groups. As discussed in Chapter 2, domain experts' knowledge developed on the basis of their experience, and education has an impact on the eye gaze pattern. In Chapter 5, it was discovered that there is difference between eye gaze pattern of the expert and nonexpert groups for the optic disc (OD) detection task. The experts' gaze fixations were concentrated on target, that is, the OD region, and the nonexperts' gazes were attracted by other regions of the fundus images as well. This chapter is dedicated to developing an approach that makes use of these differences for region labelling. The approach here identifies two regions: attractor region and distractor region.

In any target search process, the main aspect of the visual search is how the knowledge about target helps in search process. Participant's prior knowledge about the target features improves the performance and makes search efficient.

\-

* A part of this chapter has been published as poster with title "An Eye Gaze Based Approach for Labelling Regions in Fundus Retinal Images" in 19th European Conference on Eye Movements, ECEM 2017 and abstract is published in Journal of Eye Movement Research, ISSN: 1995-8692, p. 297.

According to the expert searchers, a prior knowledge of the target always has an important role. Similarly, absence of target knowledge results in slow search and hence increases the search errors.

For example, not knowing the colour of your friends' dress can make it much more difficult to find them in a crowded scene. While searching a target, the eye movements are governed toward the target (Williams, 1966, 1967). The eye movements are also guided toward both types of distractors: first those that share feature similarities with the target and second those that do not (Findlay, 1997; Motter, 1994).

Similarly, the knowledge about the distractor will also affect the search process. The presence of distractors may result in incorrect localization of target, delay in search process, and increase in search errors. If the observer is aware of features or physical properties of the distractors that differentiate them from the targets, then the search process can be improved. The search performance can be degraded by heterogeneity of distractors (Avraham et al., 2008; Nagy et al., 2005) and by replacement of old distractors with a new subset of distractors (Rosenholtz et al., 2007). The distractors with salient properties, but not sharing visual features with the targets, attract attention and trigger eye movements toward them (Theeuwes & Burger, 1998). The effects of these distractors can be minimized with practice (Geyer et al., 2008; Eckstein, 2011).

It has been understood from the discussion that identification of distractor regions is also important along with the target region. This chapter focuses on the automatic labelling of retinal images using eye gaze analysis (ALRIEGA) unit of the eye gaze–based optic disc detection (EGODD) system. In ALRIEGA unit, a novel method for identification/labelling of the target [attractor region or regions of interest (ROIs)] and distractor regions in fundus retinal images is discussed.

For image region labelling, two commonly used techniques are the following: (1) manual labelling, which is time-consuming and difficult (experienced domain experts required), and (2) automatic labelling. Many works in the literature on the automatic labelling of the target region are reported. The large-scale annotation of the web pages was carried out by Tsai et al. (2011). The annotation is based on images that share similar visual features and belong to the same semantic concept. There were a few algorithms in the literature that use the salient image region for labelling. An approach by Rowe (2002) is based on image processing. The image segmentation and low-level processing is used to find the visual focus of an image. The approach here is to link visual focus with the image caption (single object only). It has a limitation for the position and characteristics of the object. By learning a fixated image vocabulary, Duygulu et al. (2002) performed a mapping between region types and keywords supplied with the images. The method that gives local image patches as a result of over segmentation is used here. The method given by Liu et al. (2009) automatically assign labels at image level to image regions. Images used were simple with 2–3.5 labels per image. The work concluded that two images with the same label are likely to contain similar patches.

Currently, gaze information is used for analysis; for example, web pages are marked with ROI. The eye gazes were analysed based on ROIs to optimize object under examination (Castagnos et al., 2010). These ROIs were manually created. These approaches indicate that the eye-tracking data deliver reliable information about the human perception of specific image regions. In another approach, the image was classified as follows: handshake, crowd, landscape, main object in uncluttered background, and miscellaneous, by analysing common gaze trajectories (Jaimes et al., 2001). The object definition model that allows the users to specify the relation of objects in the images is given. Pasupa et al. (2009) showed the application of Support Vector Machine (SVM) algorithm and eye-tracking information to rank images. To identify the most independent image region, a method was given by Santella et al. (2006). Klami (2010) identified image regions relevant in a specific task using gaze information. The given task here is generic; the work was not aiming to identify single objects in the image. Ramanathan et al. (2010) propounded a method that used gaze data to find the seed point for the segmentation algorithm. This segmentation approach performed 10% better than that without gaze data.

There are many algorithms in the literature for automatic labelling that have been built based on visual features of the objects or based on the saliency of objects. There are certain images in which the target region is not salient but important. A human observer is required to identify such image regions. Similarly, most of the methods reported aim to identify or label only the target or ROI.

Chapter 5 showed that the experts use their knowledge and experience during the task. This prior knowledge of the experts is reflected in their eye gaze pattern and their eye gaze was guided toward the target region. So, in automatic labelling of retinal images using eye gaze analysis (ALRIEGA) unit, the expert's eye fixations were used for identifying the target regions and nonexpert's eye fixations were used for identifying distractor regions.

The ALRIEGA unit is discussed in Section 6.1. Sections 6.2 and 6.3 give the results and summary for this chapter, respectively.

6.1 Automatic Labelling of Retinal Images using Eye Gaze Analysis (ALRIEGA) System

The ALRIEGA unit aims to identify/label attractor and distractor regions. The extracted eye gaze features from the experts and nonexpert groups in eye gaze data processing and analysis (EGDPA) unit are given as input to ALRIEGA unit, as shown in Figure 6.1. The working of automatic labelling of retinal images using eye gaze analysis (ALRIEGA) unit is given in Figure 6.2.

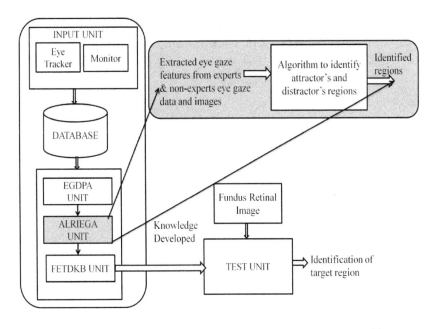

Figure 6.1 The eye gaze–based optic disc detection (EGODD) system with detailed view of automatic labelling of retinal images using eye gaze analysis (ALRIEGA) unit

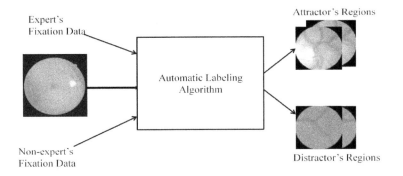

Figure 6.2 Working of automatic labelling of retinal images using eye gaze analysis (ALRIEGA) unit

In the proposed approach k-means algorithm is used for clustering. The eye gaze data are continuous data, and k-means algorithm is suitable for clustering of continuous data. The elbow method is used to ascertain the suitability of a number of clusters, as shown in Figure 6.3.

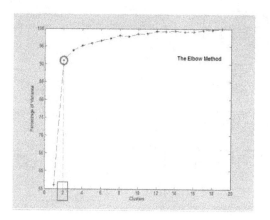

Figure 6.3 The elbow method gives the value of k as 2

As shown in Figure 6.3, the value of $k = 2$ has been found appropriate for the given data. The proposed algorithm is derived based on the value of $k = 2$. But the algorithm can be modified for various values of k based on the experimental task given and collected eye gaze data. The method for identifying attractor region is given in Figure 6.4.

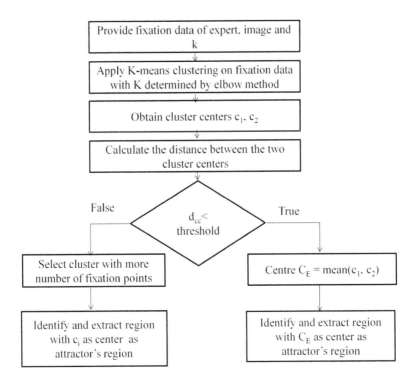

Figure 6.4 Method for identifying attractor region

The distance d_{cc} calculated is necessary because k-means algorithm can find the two clusters in the near vicinity, as shown in Figure 6.5. In the proposed algorithm, detecting the OD as one region was aimed. Thus, if the calculated distance d_{cc} is less than the threshold, the mean of the two clusters were calculated. This calculated mean is used to identify the OD region.

If the distance d_{cc} is greater than the threshold, the number of fixations in each cluster was examined. The cluster with maximum number of fixations was considered for further processing. The centre of this cluster was used as the centre for identifying the circular region, which gives attractor region. In a similar way, distractor regions were calculated with using nonexpert's eye fixation data; the method for identifying attractor region is given in Figure 6.6.

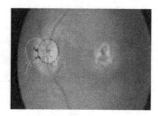

Figure 6.5 Calculated clusters from expert's fixation data

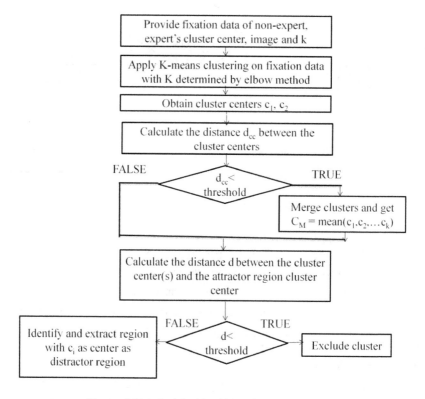

Figure 6.6 Method for identifying distractor regions

The distance is calculated between two cluster centres c_1 and c_2 for nonexpert's data. If the distance is less than threshold, the clusters are merged else the distance between these cluster centres and the attractor region cluster centre (i.e. final expert cluster centre for image n) is calculated. The purpose of this distance calculation is to check the cluster overlapping attractor region, as shown in Figure 6.7. The overlapping cluster with attractor region is shown with the green circle. For the nonexpert's fixation data, this cluster is ignored, whereas the cluster for which the distance is more is considered for further analysis. This is because by using nonexpert's eye gaze fixation data, image regions that distract attention were searched. The area that is identified with the nonexpert's fixation is called distractor region.

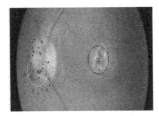

Figure 6.7 Calculated clusters from nonexpert's fixation data

6.2 Results

Attractor and distractor regions were identified for all participants from both groups. The 100 attractor regions and 250 distractor regions were identified for dataset A by processing expert's and nonexpert's fixation data. The classified attractor and distractor regions based on the algorithm are shown in Figure 6.8.

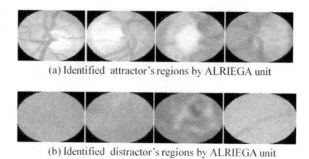

(a) Identified attractor's regions by ALRIEGA unit

(b) Identified distractor's regions by ALRIEGA unit

Figure 6.8 (a) Attractor regions, and (b) distractor regions

The detected OD region with expert's eye gaze fixations is shown in Figure 6.9. The red "X" mark indicates mean x and mean y value of the expert's fixations. The success rate for all selected images from the STARE and DRIVE datasets is 100%.

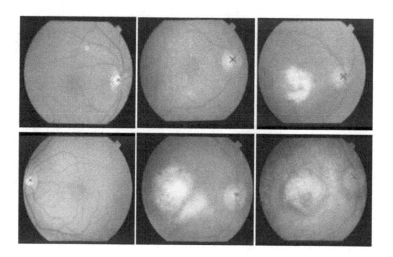

Figure 6.9 Detected OD with expert's eye gaze fixations

The performance was evaluated by measuring the average overlap between the true OD regions and the regions obtained using the proposed method, as given in the well-known technique propounded by Lalonde et al. (2001). They used an overlapping score S, which is defined to measure the common area between a true OD region T and a detected region D:

$$S = \frac{Area(T \cap D)}{Area(T \cup D)}$$

(6.1)

The average overlap of the identified attractor region by automatic labelling of retinal images using eye gaze analysis (ALRIEGA) unit and the ground truth OD region was calculated. The ground truth for the DRIVE and STARE was taken from the method by Roychowdhury et al. (2016). The average overlap of the identified attractor region by automatic labelling of retinal images using eye gaze analysis (ALRIEGA) unit and ground truths for the DRIVE dataset was 98.24% and that for the STARE dataset was 97.81%. The results of identified attractor regions were validated by an expert optometrist.

6.3 Summary

The chapter emphasizes on developing an approach for automatic labelling of the target or attractor and distractor regions using eye gaze data (ALRIEGA unit). The regions are identified by considering the effect of observer's domain expertise and knowledge on the image. Instead of analysing the observer, the approach proposed here uses observer's expertise and knowledge for identifying the regions in the image.

As discussed in Section 6.2, there are various image labelling approaches in the literature that make use of similar visual features, the salient image region, image features, and so on for region labelling. Another aspect of image labelling is using eye gaze data. The eye gaze data are used for image categorizations, ranking images, and finding seed pixels for identifying region. An attempt was made in U.S. Patent No. US8311279B2 (2012) to identify ignored regions using eye tracking. The distracting element in an image was identified in U.S. Patent No. US8929680B2 (2015).

An interesting aspect of the proposed approach is that it identifies the target region with domain expert's eye fixation data and distractor region with nonexpert's eye fixation data. Irrespective of the saliency of the image region, experts look into important regions whereas nonexperts look into the regions that attract their attention.

Despite the simplicity of the proposed approach, it works well for labelling regions in fundus retinal images. It can be further used for labelling the regions in different types of images, for example, medical images, natural images, and artificial images. Moreover, as the domain experts' knowledge and expertise is reflected from their eye gaze pattern, so in medical field, it may result in a number of exciting breakthroughs. The automatic labelling of the target regions and distractor regions using eye gaze data proposed here enhances the literature of region labelling. The image features are extracted from these identified regions for further processing, which are discussed in Chapter 7.

Chapter 7

7   FEATURE EXTRACTION AND TOP-DOWN KNOWLEDGE GENERATION[*]

In the previous chapter, the focus was on the automatic labelling of fundus retinal images into attractor and distractor regions. This labelling was based on the eye gaze fixation data collected from the expert optometrist and nonexpert groups. The expert's eye gaze fixation data were used for identification of attractor region and nonexpert eye gaze fixation data were used to identify distractor region. This chapter explains the feature extraction and top-down knowledge building (FETDKB) unit of the eye gaze-based optic disc detection (EGODD) system as, shown in Figure 7.1.

Identified attractor and distractor regions in automatic labelling of retinal images using eye gaze analysis (ALRIEGA) unit will be given as input to the feature extraction and top-down knowledge building (FETDKB) unit.

The output of the FETDKB unit is top-down (TD) knowledge, which is further used in a test unit for generation of top-down (TD) map.

----

[*]A part of this chapter was published with title "Feature extraction and selection for classification of attractor's and distractor's regions in fundus retinal images," in Proceedings of International Conference on Recent innovations in Engineering and Technologies (ICRIET-2K16), 2016.
[*] The part of this chapter has been published as poster publication with title "Top-down knowledge generation from regions in the fundus retinal images," in Grace Hopper Celebration India (GHCI) 2017. It is the **second Winner Technical Poster** in GHCI 2017.

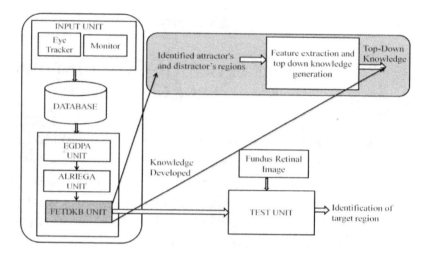

Figure 7.1 The eye gaze–based optic disc detection (EGODD) system with detailed view of feature extraction and top-down knowledge building (FETDKB) unit

The major steps involved in the feature extraction and top-down knowledge building (FETDKB) unit are feature extraction and top-down (TD) knowledge generation, which are discussed in detail in the upcoming sections. The chapter also discusses the test unit of the eye gaze–based optic disc detection (EGODD) system where the EGODD system evaluation on various standard fundus retinal datasets is explained.

The feature extraction is explained in Section 7.1. The top-down (TD) knowledge generation is discussed in Section 7.2. Test unit of the eye gaze–based optic disc detection (EGODD) system is explained in Section 7.3. Results are given in Section 7.4 followed by a summary of the chapter in Section 7.5.

7.1 Feature Extraction

Feature extraction in image processing and computer vision is a low-level image-processing operation. It gives abstraction of image information. It is generally performed as the first operation on an image. It helps to make local decision regarding whether the given type of feature is present or not at every image point. The types of features include colour, texture, shape, edges, interest points, and region of interest (ROI) points. This section discusses about the choice of features, feature extraction, and decision tree classification.

7.1.1 Choice of Features

The computation models are biologically motivated models, which helps to predict human perception (Itti & Koch, 2001; Jampani et al., 2012). The intensity, orientation and colour are three main features focused by most of the computational attention systems (Itti et al., 1998; Frintrop, 2006; Koch & Ullman, 1985). The main reasons for this choice is these features belong to the basic features proposed in psychological and biological works (Treisman & Gelade, 1980; Wolfe, 1994; Palmer, 2002) and that they are relatively easy to compute (Frintrop, 2006). This evidence from psychological and biological works forms the basis for selection of features in this research.

The perception and processing of colour starts in the retina with different types of photoreceptors. There are three types of receptors with preferences for red, green, and blue colours. Later, the processing is extended from this trichromatic architecture to the opponent processing with the colour opponents red–green and blue–yellow (Frintrop, 2006).

Thus, in the eye gaze–based optic disc detection (EGODD) system, the features such as red, green, blue, and yellow colours; the other map called colour opponency map for red–green, blue–yellow, and their complements green-red and yellow-blue; intensity; and orientation were selected for extraction.

7.1.2 Procedure for Feature Extraction

The features such as colour, intensity, and orientation were extracted from attractor and distractor regions. Along with colour feature map for red, green, blue, and yellow, the other map called colour opponency map for red-green, blue-yellow and their complements green-red and yellow-blue were extracted. The feature extraction followed the methods described in Itti et al. (1998). For each attractor and distractor region, the features were extracted using the formulas given below.

$$R = r - (g + b)/2 \tag{7.1}$$

$$G = g - (r + b)/2 \tag{7.2}$$

$$B = b - (r + g)/2 \tag{7.3}$$

$$Y = r + g - 2(|r - g| + b) \tag{7.4}$$

$$RG(c, s) = |(R(c) - G(c)) \ominus (G(s) - R(s))| \tag{7.5}$$

$$BY(c, s) = |(B(c) - Y(c)) \ominus (Y(s) - b(s))| \tag{7.6}$$

$$GR(c, s) = |(G(c) - R(c)) \ominus (R(s) - G(s))| \tag{7.7}$$

$$YB(c, s) = |Y(c) - B(c) \ominus (B(s) - Y(s))| \tag{7.8}$$

$$I = (r + g + b)/3 \tag{7.9}$$

$$I(c, s) = |I(c) \ominus I(s)| \tag{7.10}$$

$$O_{n,\alpha} = LPF[e^{(i\vec{k_\alpha} \cdot \vec{r})} L_n[x, y]] \tag{7.11}$$

where

$O_{n,\alpha}$ is the oriented image at scale n and orientation α.

$\vec{r} = x\vec{i} + y\vec{j}$, x and y are the spatial coordinates of the Laplacian image.

$\vec{k_\alpha} = \left(\frac{\pi}{2}\right)[cos\theta_\alpha \vec{i} + sin\theta_\alpha \vec{j}]$

$\theta_\alpha = \left(\frac{\pi}{n}\right)(\alpha - 1) \quad (\alpha = 1 \dots N)$

$N = 4$ (because four oriented components are used corresponding to 0°, 45°, 90°, and 135°)

The colour feature map was obtained using the input image in RGB colour space. The red, green, blue, and yellow colour channels were obtained using Equations (7.1–7.3). Each channel yields maximum response to the hue to which it is tuned, and zero response to black-and-white inputs.

For obtaining the feature map, each feature channel was subsampled into two scales of Gaussian pyramid and the centre-surround difference was obtained. Here the colour opponency maps were created by using centre-surround method. The two-level Gaussian pyramid was created, where the first level was used as the centre pixel and the second level was used as surround pixel. Initially, the image was filtered using Gaussian filter and subsampled to half its size for obtaining level one. The level-one image was again filtered and subsampled to half the size, to obtain level two. The centre-surround difference was calculated by taking the fine scale as the centre (c) and the coarse scale as the surrounding (s) and performing across scale subtraction. Across scale difference between two maps, denoted by "$\ominus$" is obtained by interpolation to the finer scale and point-by-point subtraction.

The "centre-surround" differences detect the spatial discontinuities for each feature. The centre is the pixel at level $c=2$ in the pyramid, and the surround to that pixel is at level $s=c+\delta$, with $\delta = [1,2]$.

The colour opponency maps were obtained by creating Gaussian pyramid for the red, green, blue, and yellow feature maps. The RG colour opponency maps have red regions highlighted and green regions inhibited whereas BY colour opponency map have blue regions highlighted and yellow regions inhibited. For computing colour opponency maps, the Gaussian pyramid is created for the red, green, blue, and yellow features maps obtained using Equations (7.1)–(7.4). Using Equations (7.5)–(7.8), the four-colour opponency maps were obtained.

The intensity map is created by finding the average of red, green, and blue components. After finding the average, the centre-surround difference of the intensity map is obtained for the calculation of intensity feature map. The centre-surround difference is obtained as explained for the colour feature maps (Equation 7.10).

The orientation maps are computed using oriented pyramids. Log-Gabor filters were used for obtaining the different orientation maps and implemented based on the Greenspan et al. (1994) method. The orientation pyramid consists of four pyramids, one for each orientation 0°, 45°, 90°, and 135°. The pyramid for each orientation highlights the edges having this orientation on different scales. Gabor filters are the product of a symmetric Gaussian with an oriented sinusoid and this stimulates the respective field structure of orientation-selective neurons in primary visual cortex. A Laplacian pyramid of the image is created using filter–subtract–decimate (FSD) method and each level of the pyramid is modulated with a set of oriented sign waves. Gabor filters directly give the centre-surround difference output and hence the output is directly considered for feature map (Equation 7.11).

A total of 13 features were obtained from each of attractor and distractor regions. There are four feature maps for RGBY colour features, four feature maps for red-green, blue-yellow, green-red, and yellow-blue features; one intensity feature map; and four orientation feature maps for 0°, 45°, 90°, and 135° orientations, as shown in Table 7.1. The features are extracted from all attractor and distractor regions.

Table 7.1 Number of features extracted

Features	Numbers
Colour (RGBY)	4
Colour opponency (RG, BY, GR, YB)	4
Intensity	1
Orientation map (0°, 45°, 90°, 135°)	4
Total	13

Total feature samples extracted from attractor and distractor regions were 350. Moreover, the collected samples were classified as samples from disjunctive type of images (280 samples) and samples from conjunctive type of images (70 samples). Further analysis was performed to understand how the extracted features were able to classify regions as attractor and distractor regions by applying a simple decision tree classifier. Three machine-learning models were trained using the training sets (Amudha et al., 2011). To train the decision tree classifier, a set of 70, 280, and 350 samples from conjunctive, disjunctive, and complete set, respectively, were used, as given in Table 7.2. The 10-fold cross-validation is used here.

Table 7.2 Number of samples from each set

Set	Number of Samples
Conjunctive	70
Disjunctive	280
Complete	350

Table 7.3 Classifier accuracy by classifier models for three sets

Classifier Model	Complete Set	Disjunctive Set	Conjunctive Set
J48	94.57%	95.34%	94.28%
SimpleCart	94.57%	92.47%	94.28%
LADTree	95.42%	96.05%	94.28%

The classification performance was evaluated by three decision tree models: J48, SimpleCart, and LADTree. The classifier models were evaluated for three datasets—complete set, conjunctive set, and disjunctive set, as given in Table 7.3. It is shown that maximum accuracy is 95.42% for complete set, 96.05% for disjunctive set, and 94.28% for conjunctive set. From the classification result, it is clear that, based on the extracted features, the two regions are classified with good classification accuracy.

After comparison of this result with that of the visual attention–based optic disc detection (VAODD) system given in Chapter 4, it is seen that there is an improvement in the results for complete, disjunctive, and conjunctive type of images.

In human perception theory there are two types of targets. One is conjunctive and another is disjunctive; in a search when the target and distractors are completely different, it is called disjunctive target. When the target and distractors share more than one property, a serial attention is required to locate targets. Such type of search is called a conjunctive target (as discussed in Section 3.2.2). In both disjunctive and conjunctive targets knowledge of distractors helps in identification of target. In case of visual attention based (VAODD) system only bottom up approach was used.

By investigating behavioral differences in the eye gaze patterns of expert and nonexpert groups on optic disc detection task, establishing that the gaze fixations of the experts group were concentrated on optic disc region, while those of nonexpert groups were attracted by other regions of fundus image as well. Here we identified attractor region and distractor regions. These both regions were used for classification and hence the improvement in the result.

The IK model used in the visual attention–based optic disc detection (VAODD) system works with features such as colour, intensity, and orientation. In the eye gaze–based optic disc detection (EGODD) system, similar features are extracted; however in this approach, the results are found to be improved. The classifier results here are based on the fact that only attractor and distractor regions were considered for classifications. The classification results will be affected if the complete fundus retinal image is given as input. Similarly, if this is assumed as final system, then the eye tracker is the essential hardware requirement because the device is required for identifying attractor and distractor regions.

110

So, to make system testing independent of the eye tracker device and to consider fundus retinal image as input for OD detection, the top-down (TD) knowledge is developed from the extracted features, which is discussed in Section 7.2.

7.1.3 Bottom-Up Map

The bottom-up (BU) map is drawn from the input image. Conspicuity maps are constructed by summing up the feature maps corresponding to each feature. The colour conspicuity map (CCM) is the combination of RG, BY, GR, and YB feature maps (Equations 7.5–7.8). The intensity conspicuity map (ICM) is the same as the intensity feature map (Equation 7.10). The orientation conspicuity map (OCM) is obtained by adding the feature maps for all the four orientations. To get the bottom-up (BU) map, all the conspicuity maps are summed and normalized to the range 0–255.

$$BU\ MAP = N\ (ICM + CCM + OCM)\qquad\qquad (7.12)$$

7.2 Top-Down Knowledge Generation

The feature ranking is used for generation of top-down (TD) knowledge. Many feature selection and feature-ranking methods have been proposed in the literature (e.g., Mántaras, 1991; Setiono & Liu, 1996; Sridhar et al., 1998). The feature ranking determines the importance of individual feature. Ranking methods are based on statistics, information theory, or on some functions of classifier's outputs. The attribute evaluations commonly used are information gain (IG), gain ratio, symmetrical uncertainty, relief-F, one-R, and chi-squared (χ^2).

The aim of this work was to determine the contribution made by features for discriminating between the classes. Thus, in this research, InfoGainAttributeEval with ranker search method in WEKA (Waikato Environment for Knowledge Analysis) was used for ranking the features. It evaluates the worth of a feature/attribute by measuring the IG with respect to the class.

As training dataset, 100 samples of attractor class and 250 samples of distractor class were used; each sample in both classes had 13 features. The set were given as input to WEKA. The InfoGainAttributeEval evaluates features by measuring the information gain (IG) (Equation 7.13).

$$IG \ (class, feature) = H(class) - H \ (class|feature) \qquad (7.13)$$

The InfoGainAttributeEval measures how each feature contributes in decreasing overall entropy. Entropy is commonly used in the information theory measure that characterizes the purity of an arbitrary collection of examples. It is the foundation of the IG attribute-ranking methods. The entropy of Y is

$$H \ (Y) = - \sum_{y \in Y} p(y) \log_2 (p(y)) \qquad (7.14)$$

where $p(y)$ is the marginal probability density function for the random variable Y. If the observed values of Y in the training dataset S are partitioned according to the values of a second feature X, and the entropy of Y with respect to the partitions induced by X is less than the entropy of Y before partitioning, there is a relationship between features Y and X. Then the entropy of Y after observing X is:

$$H(Y|X) = - \sum_{x \in X} p(x) \sum_{y \in Y} p(y|x) \log_2(p(y|x)) \qquad (7.15)$$

where $p(y|x)$ is the conditional probability of y given x (Novakovic et al., 2011). The output from WEKA is the ranking of the features extracted from attractor and distractor regions, as shown in Figure 7.2. Below is the list of ranked features as given in Figure 7.2

Ranked attributes:

0.585	GREEN
0.504	RG
0.409	RED
0.328	ORIENTATION-90
0.309	INTENSITY
0.293	ORIENTATION-135
0.279	ORIENTATION-45
0.279	YELLOW
0.276	YB
0.264	GR
0.243	ORIENTATION-0
0	BLUE
0	BY

The ranking here is specifically for the OD region detection, which depends on the training dataset features of the attractor class and distractor class. If the eye gaze–based optic disc detection (EGODD) system proposed here needs to be extended for other target detection application, then, based on training dataset features, the ranking will change.

The term "top-down knowledge" here indicates learning the importance of individual features extracted from attractor and distractor regions, which are identified using eye fixation data from the expert and nonexpert groups for OD detection. This top-down (TD) knowledge is used for building the top-down (TD) map.

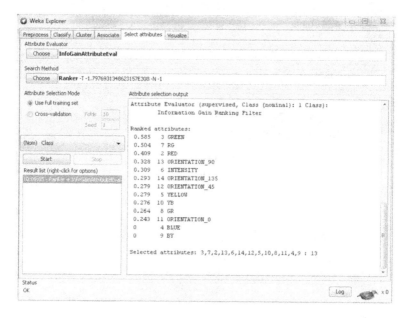

Figure 7.2 Result of InfoGainAttribute with ranker search method

7.2.1 Top-Down Map

The Fuzzy Inference System (FIS) is used in this research to compute the values for feature maps for building top-down (TD) map. The FIS is designed using the Fuzzy Toolbox in the MATLAB. The fuzzy system will assign membership values to the features according to sequence. The FIS has 13 input variables and 13 output variables representing a single pixel values, as shown in Figure 7.3. All the input and output variables have three membership functions—small, medium, and large—represented by linguistic variables, as shown in Figure 7.4.

There are 13 input variables and 13 output variables namely f_1, f_2, f_3, f_4, f_5, f_6, f_7, f_8, f_9, f_{10}, f_{11}, f_{12}, and f_{13}. The f_i' gives the output maps (with $i = 1$–13). These feature maps are obtained from the input fundus test image using feature extraction methods explained in Section 7.1.2. On the basis of top-down (TD) knowledge, the feature maps were rearranged and fed to the fuzzy system.

Table 7.4 Input features f_1–f_{13} given to fuzzy system

Input Variable	Feature
f_1	GREEN
f_2	RG
f_3	RED
f_4	ORIENTATION-90
f_5	INTENSITY
f_6	ORIENTATION-135
f_7	ORIENTATION-45
f_8	YELLOW
f_9	YB
f_{10}	GR
f_{11}	ORIENTATION-0
f_{12}	BLUE
f_{13}	BY

Based on the ranking given in Figure 7.2, f1 represents green, f2 represents RG, f3 represents red, f4 represents orientation_90, f5 represents Intensity, f6 represents orientation_135, f7 represents orientation_45, f8 represents yellow, f9 represents YB, f10 represents GR, f11 represents orientation_0, f12 represents blue, and f13 represents BY; these will be inputs given to the fuzzy system (Table 7.4).

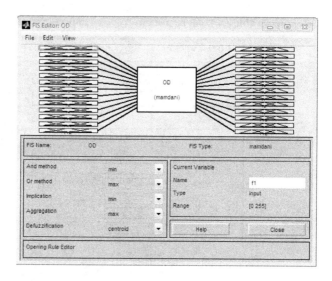

Figure 7.3 Fuzzy inference system (FIS) designed for the eye gaze–based optic disc detection (EGODD) system

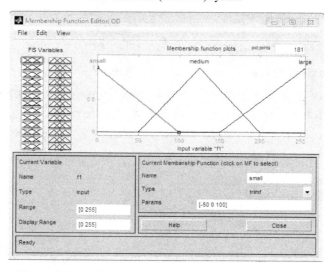

Figure 7.4 The linguistic variables and membership functions

Triangular membership functions are used as they are suitable to represent pixel value. The range of the values of the pixels is 0–255. This range is divided into three for assigning to the three membership functions. The range 0–100 belongs to

116

the membership function small; the range 50–200 belongs to the membership function medium; and the range 150–255 belongs to the membership function large.

The rules are written using if or then statements (as given in Figure 7.5). These rules are written such that output features have values based on the feature ranking given in the previous section. The feature with high ranking is given the higher weightage, that is, it has a large membership value. For example, in Figure 7.2, the green feature has a high ranking, so even though the green feature in input is small, designed FIS will assign large membership for the green feature.

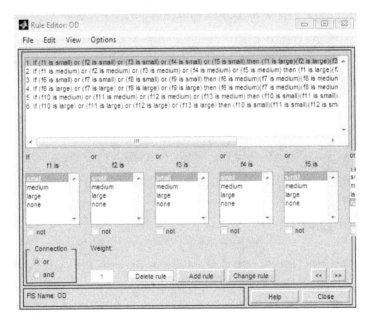

Figure 7.5 Fuzzy system rule editor

1. If (f1 is small) or (f2 is small) or (f3 is small) or (f4 is small) or (f5 is small) then (f1 is large)(f2 is large)(f3 is large)(f4 is large)(f5 is large) (1)
2. If (f1 is medium) or (f2 is medium) or (f3 is medium) or (f4 is medium) or (f5 is medium) then (f1 is large)(f2 is large)(f3 is large)(f4 is large)(f5 is large) (1)
3. If (f6 is small) or (f7 is small) or (f8 is small) or (f9 is small) then (f6 is medium)(f7 is medium)(f8 is medium)(f9 is medium) (1)
4. If (f6 is large) or (f7 is large) or (f8 is large) or (f9 is large) then (f6 is medium)(f7 is medium)(f8 is medium)(f9 is medium) (1)
5. If (f10 is medium) or (f11 is medium) or (f12 is medium) or (f13 is medium) then (f10 is small)(f11 is small)(f12 is small)(f13 is small) (1)
6. If (f10 is large) or (f11 is large) or (f12 is large) or (f13 is large) then (f10 is small)(f11 is small)(f12 is small)(f13 is small) (1)

Figure 7.6 Fuzzy rules

117

The first five features in input are assigned with large values; the next four features in the input are assigned with medium values; and the last four features in the input are assigned with small values (Figure 7.6). The fuzzy rules are written such a way that the excitation is given to the target (i.e., optic disc) region while the other parts of the image are inhibited.

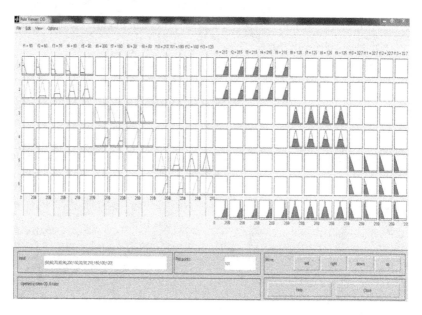

Figure 7.7 The Rule Viewer of the Fuzzy Inference system used in eye gaze–based optic disc detection (EGODD)

The Rule viewer of the Fuzzy system is shown in Figure 7.7, with 13 input variables and 13 output variables. As shown in the figure, for a sample input set with 13 features ([50 60 70 80 90 200 180 30 50 210 180 100 120]) output values for 13 maps are assigned. In this case, the first five inputs have assigned a large membership value in output maps. Similarly, next four inputs have been assigned medium membership value and the last four values in input have been assigned small membership value. The top-down (TD) map is created by finding the difference between output maps (Equation 7.16).

TD MAP = Differnce of (output_maps)

(7.16)

7.3 Test Unit

The working of test unit of the eye gaze–based optic disc detection (EGODD) system is shown in Figure 7.8. This unit takes fundus retinal image as input. It calculates two maps; bottom-up (BU) map and top-down (TD) map. The BU map is built from extracted features (Section 7.1) and TD map is calculated from the knowledge gained from ranking the features (Section 7.2).

The step include are the following:

1. Read the input test image
2. Calculate bottom-up (BU) map
3. Calculate top-down (TD) map
4. Calculate combined map
   Combined map = BU map + TD map
5. Identify the most salient region

The most salient region is detected using the region-growing method. It is the pixel-based region-growing method in which the initial seed point is given as input. The pixel having maximum value in the combined map is selected as the seed pixel. This approach examines neighbouring pixels of initial seed point and determines whether the pixel neighbours should be added to the region.

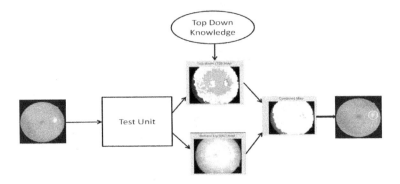

Figure 7.8 Working of test unit in the eye gaze–based optic disc detection (EGODD) system

The GUI (graphical user interface) created for the eye gaze–based optic disc detection (EGODD) system is shown in Figure 7.9, and Figure 7.10 shows how the EGODD system identifies the OD region. Figure 7.11 shows the examples of the calculated bottom-up (BU), top-down (TD), and combined maps for input fundus retinal image.

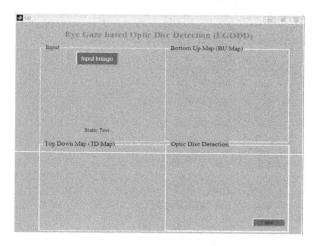

Figure 7.9 Graphical user interface of the eye gaze–based optic disc detection (EGODD) system

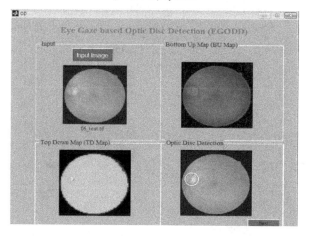

Figure 7.10 Example of fundus retinal image given as input to the eye gaze–based optic disc detection (EGODD) system

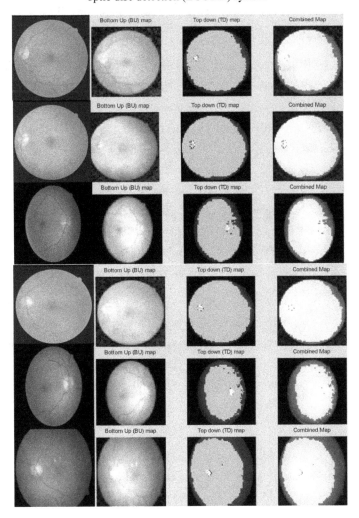

Figure 7.11 (From leftmost) Original image, bottom-up (BU) map, top-down (TD) map, and combined map generated by the eye gaze–based optic disc detection (EGODD) system

7.4 Eye Gaze–based Optic Disc Detection (EGODD) System Validation

The eye gaze–based optic disc detection (EGODD) system is validated using various parameters such as success rate, average hit number, number of first hits, and overlapping score. The hit number on image I for target t is the rank of the focus that hits the target in the order of the saliency. For example, if the second focus is on the target, the hit number is 2. The lower the hit number, the better the performance. The average hit number for the dataset is the arithmetic mean of the hit numbers of all images. The average hit number is computed for each dataset separately, as shown in Table 7.5. The number of first hits for different datasets was also computed. The number is converted into percentage so that comparison becomes easy for different datasets with different number of images. The average overlap is calculated as given in Chapter 6 (Equation 6.1).

The validation of the eye gaze–based optic disc detection (EGODD) system is carried out in two phases. In first phase, the system is tested using five standard fundus retinal datasets. Here, the system was validated based on success rate, average hit number, and number of first hits. In the first testing phase, the top-down (TD) knowledge generated using 100 attractor regions and 250 distractor regions are used.

In the second testing phase, the eye gaze–based optic disc detection (EGODD) system is evaluated using additional eye gaze data. Here, the system is tested on seven standard fundus retinal datasets. The eye gaze–based optic disc detection (EGODD) system is validated based on success rate, average hit number, number of first hits, and average overlap. In the second testing phase, the top-down (TD) knowledge generated using 469 attractor regions and 986 distractor regions are used.

The results of the eye gaze–based optic disc detection (EGODD) system were compared with those of the visual attention–based optic disc detection (VAODD) system (Chapter 4) for the STARE standard fundus retinal dataset. Similarly, the eye gaze–based optic disc detection (EGODD) system performance was tested for disjunctive and conjunctive type of images obtained from various datasets.

7.4.1 Testing of Eye Gaze–based Optic Disc Detection (EGODD) System: Phase One

In phase one, the dataset A is used as stimulus images for eye gaze data collection from two groups. The eye gaze–based optic disc detection (EGODD) system proposed here yields 95% and 97.5% success rates for the DRIVE and INSPIRE datasets, respectively. For the High Resolution Fundus Images, STARE, and DIARETDB0 datasets, the EGODD system yielded, respectively, 91.48%, 72.83%, and 88.46% success rates, as given in Table 7.5. The table also gives average hit numbers and percentage of number of first hits for five datasets (DRIVE, STARE, INSPIRE, High Resolution Fundus Images, and DIARETDB0).

Table 7.5 Results of the eye gaze–based optic disc detection (EGODD) system for various standard datasets

Datasets	Success Rates (%)	Avg. Hit Numbers	Number of First Hits (%)
DRIVE (40 Images)	95	1.81	65.78
INSPIRE (40 Images)	97.5	2.79	56
High Resolution Fundus Images (45 images)	91.48	1.81	65.11
DIARETDB0 (130 images)	88.46	1.64	83.47
STARE (81 images)	72.83	3.38	37.28

7.4.2 Testing of Eye Gaze–based Optic Disc detection (EGODD) System: Phase Two

Here, the eye gaze–based optic disc detection (EGODD) system was evaluated with additional eye gaze data collected from four expert optometrist and eight nonexpert groups. A total of 95 fundus images were used as stimulus images for eye gaze data collection. In the phase two, dataset B was used as stimulus images for eye gaze data collection from two groups. Again complete procedure for data collection was repeated. The data were collected using SMI Red-m eye tracker device.

The automatic labelling of the regions in fundus retinal images was carried out, as discussed in automatic labelling of retinal images using eye gaze analysis (ALRIEGA) unit of the eye gaze–based optic disc detection (EGODD) system (Chapter 6). The 369 attractor regions and 736 distractor regions were identified using eye fixation data from experts and nonexperts, respectively. The feature ranking was again carried out for 469 attractor regions and 986 distractor regions samples. The top-down (TD) knowledge was generated according to a new ranking. The top-down (TD) map was calculated based on this new top-down (TD) knowledge using fuzzy system. The test unit procedure was repeated for all images in each dataset. The performance of the eye gaze–based optic disc detection (EGODD) system was evaluated using two measures: success rate and average overlap. The success rate of the EGODD system for different fundus retinal images datasets is shown in Table 7.6.

The eye gaze–based optic disc detection (EGODD) system is able to detect OD with more than 90% success rate except the STARE dataset. No sample from the DRIONS-DB and ONHSD dataset is used as stimulus image for eye gaze data collection, however the EGODD system achieved, respectively, 98.2 and 91.9 success rates.

Table 7.6 Results of the eye gaze–based optic disc detection (EGODD) system
for various standard datasets (with new ranking)

Datasets	Success Rates (%)	Avg. Hit Numbers	Number of First Hits (%)
DRIVE (40 Images)	100	1.6	80
DRIONS-DB (110 images)	98.2	1.0	98.1
INSPIRE (40 Images)	97.5	1.9	79
High Resolution Fundus Images (45 images)	100	3.2	57.5
DIARETDB0 (130 images)	96.9	1.5	89.5
ONHSD (99 images)	91.9	1.2	93.4
STARE (81 images)	81.4	3.1	30.8

Table 7.6 also shows the average hit number and number of first hits for all the datasets. The results were further analysed for conjunctive type of images and disjunctive type of images for the STARE dataset and compared with those obtained from the visual attention–based optic disc detection (VAODD) system (Table 7.7).

Table 7.7 Comparison between the visual attention–based optic disc detection (VAODD) and eye gaze–based optic disc detection (EGODD) methods for the STARE dataset

Dataset	Visual Attention-based Optic Disc Detection (VAODD)			Eye Gaze-based Optic Disc Detection (EGODD)		
	Success rate	Conjunctive type of images	Disjunctive type of images	Success rate	Conjunctive type of images	Disjunctive type of images
STARE	74.07%	50%	86.79%	81.48%	82.14%	81.13%

As given in Table 7.7, the eye gaze–based optic disc detection (EGODD) system performs better than the visual attention–based optic disc detection (VAODD) system for OD detection. The success rate was 74.07% for the VAODD, which was improved to 81.48% in the eye gaze–based optic disc detection (EGODD) system. Similarly, the OD detection was 50% for conjunctive type of images, which was improved to 82.14% in the EGODD system. But here there was a decrease in performance for disjunctive type of images in the EGODD system. The reason behind that is for some images in the STARE dataset, the OD region was not visible in the images (Figure 7.12), for such images the EGODD system failed to identify OD regions.

The eye gaze–based optic disc detection (EGODD) system performance was tested for disjunctive and conjunctive type of images from various datasets, as shown in Figure 7.13. It is observed that the eye gaze–based optic disc detection (EGODD) system identifies target, that is, the OD region for disjunctive and conjunctive type of images efficiently.

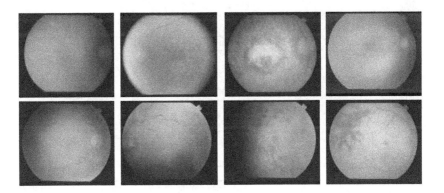

Figure 7.12 Examples of images from the STARE dataset for which the eye gaze–based optic disc detection (EGODD) system fails

Results

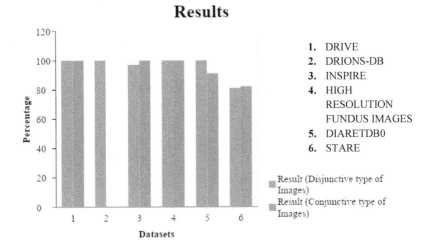

1. DRIVE
2. DRIONS-DB
3. INSPIRE
4. HIGH RESOLUTION FUNDUS IMAGES
5. DIARETDB0
6. STARE

Figure 7.13 Result of the eye gaze–based optic disc detection (EGODD) system for disjunctive and conjunctive type of images from various datasets

The results of the comparison between existing OD methods and the eye gaze–based optic disc detection (EGODD) system are given in Table 7.8. The EGODD system performs better for most of the datasets.

Table 7.8 Comparison of the proposed eye gaze–based optic disc detection (EGODD) system with existing systems on different datasets

Sr. No.	Datasets	Existing Systems' Performance Reported (%)		Proposed EGODD System Performance (%)
1	DRIVE (40 images)	Aggarwal and Khare (2014)	100	100
		Dehghani et al. (2012)	100	
		Mendonça et al. (2013)	100	
		Godse and Bormane (2013)	100	
		Welfer et al. (2013)	100	
		Wang et al. (2015)	100	
		Sinha and Babu (2012)	95	
		Ramakanth and Babu (2012)	100	
2	INSPIRE (40 images)	Muntasa et al. (2015)	81.6	97.5
3	High Resolution Fundus Images (45 images)	Khalid et al. (2014)	93.7	100
4	DIRECTDB0 (130 images)	Godse and Bormane (2013)	96.1	96.9
		Wang et al. (2015)	97.7	
		Devasia et al. (2014)	96.9	
		Sinha and Babu (2012)	96.9	
		Ramakanth and Babu (2012)	98.4	
5	STARE (81 images)	Wisaeng et al. (2014)	91.3	81.4
		Mithun et al. (2014)	91.3	
		Dehghani et al. (2012)	91	
		Reza and Ahmad (2015)	87.6	
		Lu and Lim (2011)	96.3	
		Ramakanth and Babu (2012)	93.8	
6	DRIONS-DB (110 images)	Pradhepa et al. (2015)	54.5	98.2
		Devasia et al. (2014)	95.4	
		Claro et al. (2016)	94.5	

The average overlap obtained by the eye gaze–based optic disc detection (EGODD) system and the existing system for the DRIVE, DIRECTDB 0, STARE, DRIONS-DB, and ONHSD datasets are given in Table 7.9. It has been clear from the result that the eye gaze–based optic disc detection (EGODD) system achieved an excellent average overlap.

Table 7.9 Comparison of overlapping score of the proposed eye gaze–based optic disc detection (EGODD) system with existing systems on different datasets

Methods	DRIVE (%)	DIRECTDB 0 (%)	STARE (%)	DRIONS-DB (%)	ONHSD (%)
Welfer et al. (2013)	42.54	-	-	-	-
Sopharak et al. (2008)	16.88	-	-	-	-
Kande et al. (2008)	29.66	-	-	-	-
Lupascu et al. (2008)	40.01	-	-	-	-
Wang et al. (2015)	88.17	89.06	-	-	-
Wisaeng et al. (2014)	-	-	91.35	-	-
Tjandrasa et al. (2012)	75.56 (30 images)	-	-	-	-
Girard et al., (2016)	-	-	-	-	84
Dashtbozorg et al., (2015)	-	-	-	-	83
Proposed EGODD system	96.72	96.48	95.93	97.13	95.75

The ground truths for the DRIVE, STARE, and DIRECTDB 0 were taken from Roychowdhury et al. (2016) and those for the DRIONS-DB and ONHSD were taken from Carmona et al. (2008) and Lowell et al. (2004). The average overlap for other existing system was taken from Wang et al. (2015).

7.5 Summary

The feature extraction and top-down (TD) knowledge generation have been discussed. The human perception concepts were taken into account for feature selection. Generation of top-down (TD) knowledge from eye gaze pattern added a new edge in the research. The fuzzy-based system is used for creating the top-down (TD) map. The OD region in test image was detected using bottom-up (BU) and top-down (TD) maps. It is observed that the eye gaze–based optic disc detection (EGODD) system performance is improved in testing phase two. This indicates that adding more experts and stimulus images in the learning of the system improves performance of the system. The eye gaze–based optic disc detection (EGODD) system is evaluated using seven standard datasets.

CHAPTER 8

8 CONCLUSION

Eye tracking has been used in research fields for a quite long time. However, most of the research works were carried out to compare and correlate the behaviour difference of two groups of eye gaze pattern. The thesis investigates on the need to design a system which bridges the gap between the vision and the brain. It aims to utilise the eye gaze pattern of the domain experts' and incorporates their experience through eye gaze features to identify target regions. The research is required to understand how the domain experts' experience can be used for designing a system.

Nevertheless, one of the key issues in this field is that there are not many research evidences that consider the eye tracking for target detection and thesis addresses the issue with assuming the target to be optic disc (OD) detection. The working goal throughout the thesis is to develop an eye gaze–based optic disc detection (EGODD) system. In Chapter 2, the concept underlying eye tracking and different eye movements is discussed. A survey on the use of eye tracking is given. In Chapter 3, OD detection is introduced followed by detailed survey on different OD detection methods. The identified research gaps in field of eye tracking and OD detection are highlighted.

In Chapter 4, the applicability of bottom-up (BU) visual attention model for OD detection is investigated. It is observed that only BU approach is not sufficient for OD detection. Thus, in Chapter 5, an EGODD system is introduced, which combines bottom-up (BU) and top-down (TD) approaches. The eye gaze data collection and processing is explained. The chapter also compares eye gaze pattern of the expert and nonexpert groups, which is found to be different.

The automatic labelling algorithms for identification of attractor region and distractor region are introduced in Chapter 6. The algorithms use expert's eye

131

gaze for identification of attractor regions and nonexpert's eye gaze to identify distractor regions. In Chapter 7, feature extraction from attractor and distractor regions is explained and the top-down (TD) knowledge generation is discussed. The eye gaze–based optic disc detection (EGODD) system evaluation for OD detection is also discussed.

The salient features of the proposed OD detection system can be summarized as follows. Initially, applicability of visual attention model for OD detection is investigated to understand how human perception concepts work for OD detection. It is generally a known fact that bottom-up (BU) approach does not perform well for target detection applications such as OD detection. The top-down (TD) approach has to be incorporated in the system along with the bottom-up (BU) approach to increase the performance. Thus, the top-down (TD) approach is incorporated in the form of TD knowledge generated from the eye gaze data collected by the expert and nonexpert groups.

The categorization of the images into two different categories of attractor and distractor regions using eye gaze data adds a new research direction.

The advantage of the eye gaze–based optic disc detection (EGODD) system is that it can be deployed without the need of eye-tracking equipment. It is designed in such a way that its test phase works independent of the eye tracker.

The system inherits the main advantage of the human visual perception concept and knowledge developed from expert's eye gaze pattern. It is evaluated for OD detection but is generally applicable to every target detection application.

The proposed work has been appreciated for its novelty and the system for detecting OD in fundus retinal images using eye tracking geared toward improving the state-of-the-art technology in OD detection and eye tracking.

8.1 Major Research Contributions

The major thesis contributions are given as below:

- Understanding of how human visual perception works on fundus images for OD detection, in particular how the bottom-up (BU) computational model works for OD detection. Retinal images are categorized as disjunctive, where the optic disc is also the most salient region, or conjunctive, where the optic disc is one of several salient regions. It is shown via experiments that for disjunctive images, BU attention-based models work quite well whereas for conjunctive images, their performance is poor.

- The behavioural difference in the eye gaze patterns of the expert and nonexpert groups on the optic disc detection task is investigated. It is observed that the eye gaze fixations of the expert group were concentrated on the optic disc region whereas those of the nonexpert group were attracted by other regions of the fundus images as well.

- A novel method has been developed for identifying the two regions, namely attractor region and distractor region, in retinal images. The attractor and distractor datasets are classified by extracting features from both regions.

- The ranking of individual features extracted from attractor and distractor regions is identified and an integrated system that incorporates bottom-up (BU) and top-down (TD) approaches for OD detection is developed. The proposed eye gaze–based optic disc detection (EGODD) system has been validated across various models for its performance.

8.2 Limitations and Future Work

The limitations of proposed research work are inherited from the human attention system. General human errors are possible in data collection procedure. As the research is based on the eye tracking data collected from the participants. During the data collection it is assumed that participants are attentive, mindful and conscious while doing the task. There is chance of human error. For ex, for the small amount of time participants may not be attentive, in this case the collected eye gaze data is not useful.

Although the results presented here have shown the effectiveness of the proposed system, there is still a lot of scope for improvement. The thesis opens various research issues system design can be improved by increasing the number of images and domain experts in the learning phase. Various other eye gaze measures, such as saccadic amplitude, duration, and peak velocity, can be incorporated in the system.

Since the contribution of the thesis proposed is more towards integrating eye tracking data as a top down knowledge so that the target can be easily detected. The extension of a time series eye tracking data into a deep learning architecture for the specific use case addressed in the thesis, is quite feasible recently since eye trackers have become affordable, which paved way for massive dataset creation. Hence this can be a promising future scope for the current work where deep learning as a machine learning can be integrated to the existing EGODD system. Similarly, the dataset also can be further extended thus applying the deep learning algorithm will be feasible.

The system can be tuned for different medical anomaly detection applications in various medical image modalities such as CT images, MRI, ultrasound, PET, and X-ray images. It can make use of the knowledge of experts from the respective domains.

This research is based on the anatomy structural part of human eye, that is, OD. The use of eye tracking to identify other pathological tissues in the fundus retinal image is yet to be addressed. Further investigation is needed on understanding the use of the expert's eye gaze pattern for detecting these tissues.

CPSIA information can be obtained
at www.ICGtesting.com
Printed in the USA
LVHW052129301222
736235LV00034B/1256